Psilocybin Mushroom Cultivation

The Complete Guide to Grow Indoor and Outdoor your Magic Mushrooms. Discover safe use and after-effects of Psychedelics Mushroom and How Hallucinogenic Plant Works

Pablo Medicine

Legal & Disclaimer

The information contained in this book and its contents is not designed to replace or take the place of any form of medical or professional advice; and is not meant to replace the need for independent medical, financial, legal or other professional advice or services, as may be required. The content and information in this book has been provided for educational and entertainment purposes only.

The content and information contained in this book has been compiled from sources deemed reliable, and it is accurate to the best of the Author's knowledge, information and belief. However, the Author cannot guarantee its accuracy and validity and cannot be held liable for any errors and/or omissions. Further, changes are periodically made to this book as and when needed. Where appropriate and/or necessary, you must consult a professional (including but not limited to your doctor, attorney, financial advisor or such other professional advisor) before using any of the suggested remedies, techniques, or information in this book.

Upon using the contents and information contained in this book, you agree to hold harmless the Author from and against any damages, costs, and expenses, including any legal fees potentially resulting from the application of any of the information provided by this book. This disclaimer applies to any loss, damages or injury caused by the use and application, whether directly or indirectly, of any advice or information presented, whether for breach of contract, tort, negligence, personal injury, criminal intent, or under any other cause of action.

You agree to accept all risks of using the information presented inside this book.

You agree that by continuing to read this book, where appropriate and/or necessary, you shall consult a professional (including but not limited to your doctor, attorney, or financial advisor or such other advisor as needed) before using any of the suggested remedies, techniques, or information in this book.

Table of Contents

Introduction

More and more, we hear how we supplement our daily diet with mushrooms. There is much confusion about what mushrooms are, what to eat when to eat them, and what is so good for them with us. People who study it are called mycologists. First, the question is, is a mushroom a vegetable? This is one of those questions that are not easy to answer. Remember, these are mushrooms that have been bred from mycelium. Mostly, they fall into the category of vegetable varieties, which are plants. A vegetable is considered in the culinary world as an "edible part of a plant with a savory taste." The attracting point about mushrooms is that they absorb and concentrate more than many other "plants" on what they have grown. But depending on where it is grown, it can work the other way round and be a bad thing. For example, mushrooms can concentrate on what's in the water that feeds them. Good clean water, great; However, contaminated or pesticide-contaminated water is drawn into the mushroom in the same manner. Mushrooms are an excellent example of one of the places where you should pay attention to organic quality. A good reason to grow yourself, so that you can control the water, but also the medium in which the spores grow. Mushrooms start from a spore that is so small and you might actually not see it grow unlike a seed that you can collect and sprinkle on your growth medium; The spore seems invisible. While a seed has chlorophyll and can germinate and start the growth process, a spore does not. Instead, it must have a growth medium that nourishes it and starts its growth process.

Some of the options for mushroom culture include straw, wood shavings, sawdust, wood shells, cardboard, corncob, or even composted manure. While you can buy spores, it's best to start spawning instead. Once you are an experienced veteran who grows his own mushrooms, you may want to start with the spores. Spawn is the next stage of spores, and if they have formed a root-like, pure mycelium, this is the beginning of your fungus. Technically, only the spawn can produce mushrooms under certain conditions. However, you want to add it to a nutrient medium to maintain the health of the plant and the products you want to eat. They can become moist, in dry flakes, or in dry brick form. Moist is ready to go, use it immediately, and the dry versions are designed to be used when you are ready or when the conditions are right.

Although it is important for the success of your healthy mushrooms, which does not need much water, in fact, too much water will kill it. Instead of "pouring" the seeds in your garden, you want to focus more on spraying. Some people even prefer to start with a piece of material over the spawn and just let this material moisten. Again by fogging, not by over-pouring. Traditionally, growing mushrooms indoors is a faster process, but it can also be done outdoors. Some people prefer to build a "mushroom house" that resembles a chicken coop or a small greenhouse. Mushrooms are best for dark and cool, humid environments. A cellar is, therefore, often an option. However, make sure that it is not drafts, direct heat sources (or alternating current), i.e. the sunlight. Enoki can tolerate even lower temperatures of up to 45 degrees Fahrenheit. Some even prefer to grow their mushrooms in the kitchen, in the cupboard under the sink. Depending on the temperature, you can grow mushrooms all year round and prepare your dishes, salads, and sauces fresh.

Just a piece of advice for you; do not collect wild mushrooms and do not eat them unless you know how to identify them. Wild mushrooms can make you sick, and they can kill you too. The majority of the deaths reported by the consumption of wild mushrooms are from amatoxins. There are no cure or antidote for amatoxin. Immediately, when you noticed you'd eaten the wild mushroom you have is not to be late, go to the hospital quickly, and try to remove as much venom from you as possible before your body absorbs it. Mushroom picking can be a lot of fun and is pretty straightforward. It is also very, very safe if you use trustworthy and reliable channels and do not try to create your program. Mushrooms are known for their nutritional and medicinal benefits and can be an excellent part of your "right" food.

Magic Mushroom fans play with them. Doctors study them. Cooks around the world cook mostly with mushrooms. They mostly appear overnight, disappear just as fast, and leave no trace of their visit. Students around the world are called mycologists, and now the fungus is considered a potential treatment for cancer, PTSD post-traumatic stress disorder, and some mental disorders. Mushrooms, sometimes called toadstools, are fleshy mushroom bodies that grow above ground or a food source.

Mushrooms are as a result of the growth of a fungus minus chlorophyll. These are living things that can neither be classified as plants nor as animals. Mushrooms are a traditional delicacy in Japan, Korea, and China and are valued for their taste as well as their health benefits. They have been grown in the mountainous regions of Asia using traditional techniques for more than a thousand years. During autumn, mushrooms appear between the leaves that fall from the trees and feel fresh and soft. Mushrooms are low in sodium, contain about 80 to 90 percent water and are very low in calories. A serving of mushrooms also provides about 20 to 40 percent of the daily value of copper, a mineral with cardiovascular protective properties. Selenium is an antioxidant that, together with Vitamin E, protects cells from the harmful effects of free radicals in the blood. It has been found that selenium reduces the risk of prostate cancer by 65%.

They are very nutritious and are great for treating nutritional problems as they are high in vitamins A, E and C. These mushrooms also contain lentinan, a proven cure for cancer. Some mushrooms have anti-inflammatory properties that can be very helpful in combating certain diseases in the future. Mushrooms are an excellent source of minerals that helps reduce high blood pressure and reduce the risk of stroke. Potassium keeps you from cramping for prolonged periods of exercise. A medium-sized Portabella mushroom has even more potassium than a banana or a glass of orange juice. The mushrooms are well-suited to the diet of pregnant women and children because they are rich in phosphorus, a substance that promotes bone mineralization. They also contain a lot of iodine, which is involved in growth processes. They are mineral that is essential for the proper functioning of the thyroid, which regulates metabolism. They have a little sodium and fat, and 8 to 10 percent of the dry weight of fiber. So mushrooms are good to eat if you are trying to lose more weight and they keep you regular. Mushrooms have a higher protein content than normal vegetables and are also rich in puritan, which turns the body into uric acid. People with gout, kidney stones, and hyperuricemia should, therefore, limit their consumption. Mushrooms are a very rich source of riboflavin and niacin. So the moral of the story is to add a few mushrooms to your salads, soups, and meals.

Chapter 1

Hallucinogenic (Psilocybin) Mushrooms

Psilocybin is a psychedelic drug that works by enacting serotonin receptors, most often in the prefrontal cortex. This part of the brain influences mood, discernment, and perception.

Psychedelic drugs work in other regions of the brain that regulate arousal and panic reactions. Psilocybin doesn't always cause active visual or auditory hallucinations. Instead, it mutilates how some people that use the tranquilize perceive objects and people already in their condition.

The quantity of the medicate, past experiences, and expectations of how the experience will take shape can all impact the effects of psilocybin.

After the gut ingests and consumes psilocybin, the body converts it to psilocyn. The hallucinogenic impacts of psilocybin usually happen within 30 minutes of ingestion and last between 4 and 6 hours.

In some individuals, the changes in sensory recognition and the underlying patterns of thoughts can last for a very long time.

Psilocybin containing Mushrooms is usually tan, brown, and small, and they are often regarded by some people in the wild as botch mushrooms containing psilocybin for any number of other mushrooms that are poisonous.

People ordinarily consume psilocybin as a fermented tea or prepare it with nourishment to veil its unpleasant taste in the mouth. Dried Mushrooms are crushed by manufacturers into powders and prepared in capsule forms, while some specific people consume these mushrooms meal with chocolate.

Psilocybin is delegated a Schedule I tranquilize, which means that it has a high potential for misuse and has no currently accepted therapeutic use in treatment in the United States.

Although certain societies have known to use the stimulating properties of some mushrooms for centuries, psilocybin was first secluded in 1958 by Dr. Albert Hofmann, who likewise discovered lysergic corrosive diethylamide (LSD).

Therapeutic Use

In the material above, I've offered some details as to how psilocybin and psychedelics, in general, can be used therapeutically. Testing of psilocybin by the medical community is still in its infancy, as laws have only begun to allow limited investigation within the last decade. The medical community is currently exploring its medical uses for a number of conditions. These include depression, addiction, PTSD, cluster headaches and migraines, OCD, and mood and anxiety disorders. Results thus far have been promising in each of these areas.

It's worth mentioning that initial results suggest psilocybin is far more effective in the treatment of depression than anything currently accepted for medical use. Results come more quickly and tend to be longer lasting than other drugs on the market. In addition, unlike these other drugs, patients using psilocybin for treatment of depression do not need to be continuously medicated for the treatment to be effective. In addition, initial research into the use of psilocybin treatment for addiction is more promising by far than any form of treatment thus far discovered.

Psilocybin also has great potential for emotional healing. PTSD and mood and anxiety disorder are just a few of the conditions that have been responsive to psilocybin therapy. Similar studies have shown that psilocybin has been effective at significantly reducing the emotional pain associated with social rejection.

There is no doubt that further studies will show the profound benefits of psilocybin and other psychedelics for treating trauma and all forms of emotional healing. Given the deep impact of emotion on every aspect of our lives, this suggests that psychedelics may be the single most powerful healing tool available to us.

It's noteworthy that a new research division has recently been set up and funded in the Psychiatric Department of the John Hopkins Hospital in the USA, specifically to look at the potential therapeutic effects of psychedelics–and especially psilocybin mushrooms and cannabis.

In the meantime, some relatively recent research undertaken by Dr Griffiths et al from John Hopkins University[2], is interesting and may provide some guidelines about the dosages you choose for yourself. This research helps to explain why, although it is impossible to overdose on mushrooms from a toxicity point of view and they are not addictive, it is necessary to exercise caution because of the intensity of the effects you may experience.

Griffiths et al were looking at possible therapeutic uses for psilocybin, especially for depression and PTSD, in view of its reported long-term positive effects.

They administered varying strengths of psilocybin to 30 volunteers in one study and followed it up with a similar study with 18 volunteers a few years later. They used dosages of 5, 10, 20 and 30mg psilocybin per 70kg body weight of the volunteer, administered either in increasing or decreasing dosages, and at a rate of about once per month. On average this would translate to about 0.8g, 1.6g, 3.2g and 4.8g of dried P cubensis (and matches our description of light, medium, strong and "heroic" doses given earlier).

Some of their findings are useful:

Doses of 20mg and 30mg produced a mystical experience for 72% of the group (this would be 3.2g and 4.8g in our P. cubensis calculation).

One month and even 14 months after these higher dosages, participants rated the experience as having had noteworthy personal and spiritual significance. Up to 65% also reported sustained positive changes in attitude, mood and behavior after 30mg. The 20mg group had similar results, with 60% reporting sustained positive changes.

Those who had had the ascending doses (i.e. starting low and getting stronger) reported the most positive results. This result was not the same as other research, which suggests that an immediate very strong experience might have long-term positive therapeutic results.

Those who monitored and recorded the sessions observed that most reactions increased with the increasing dosage[3]. For example, the chance of the participant crying increased with the dosage; arousal, distance from ordinary reality and happiness were highest at the 30mg dosage. However, interestingly, the highest level of peace/harmony was at the 20mg level.

Also, the researchers found that the 30mg dose gave rise to some unpleasant outcomes.

It was the only level where monitors reported significant paranoid thinking.

86% of the participants experienced extreme fearfulness, and an average time of about 11 minutes of strong anxiety. By comparison, at the 20mg level, only 14% experienced extreme fearfulness, with only 2 minutes of extreme anxiety. At 10mg, there was no fearfulness and only 1 minute of strong anxiety.

So, it would seem wise to start with low dosages, with 20mg being the most effective and carefully consider your chances of having a bad trip if you try very high dosages.

Personal Growth

While therapeutic benefits focus more on the use of psilocybin and other psychedelic compounds for healing, there may be huge benefits for healthy individuals as well. This is an exciting area of study, as it may provide a key for enhancing our capacity for healthy functioning on numerous levels. Therapeutic studies suggest that psilocybin can reduce the impact of negative states like social anxiety, distraction, and lack of motivation. At the same time, positive mental resources like creativity, cognitive function, and productivity have been enhanced through psilocybin use.

On a biological level, psilocybin has been shown to stimulate the growth of new brain cells and facilitate learning. Psilocin, the bioactive metabolite of psilocybin, stimulates the 5-HT2A serotonin receptors in the prefrontal cortex. This has two immediate biological effects. The first is an increased production of Brain Derived Neurotropic Factor (BDNF). Essentially, this stimulates the growth of neurons and neural connections and the activity of these neurons. At the same time, the brain produces more glutamate, a neurotransmitter responsible for learning, memory, and cognition.

With regard to global brain function, psilocybin dampens the activity of the Default Mode Network (DMN). This is a portion of the brain associated with a variety of mental activities including self-reflection, daydreaming, and thoughts of the past or future. When the activity of the DMN is dampened, it is easier for the brain to form new and different neural connections. This means learning new activities and information.

To put this into perspective, consider the act of concentration. Effective concentration requires present moment awareness. Thoughts of the past or future, excessive self-reflection, and daydreaming are dilutions of present moment awareness. They are processes that interfere with present moment awareness. Though these activities have their place, the DMN is often overactive, resulting in excessive self-analysis and counterproductive attention to memories or future possibilities. When the DMN has the volume turned down, the mind becomes more capable of focus and concentration, allowing us to be more productive and to learn new things more quickly and effectively.

Psilocybin also increases global neural function. In typical waking states, many parts of the brain operate more or less independently from one another. Psilocybin causes these parts of the brain to synchronize with one another, allowing more of the brain to operate as a whole rather than a collection of parts. The communication between these various regions is strengthened, and the linkages formed during the trip tend to persist even after the psychedelic experience has ended. In the process, the brain is "rebooted." It is reprogrammed and the neural activity is significantly reorganized.

Despite the advances of medical science, we still know very little about the brain compared to what is left to be discovered. Because of this, we cannot conclusively determine the impact of this reorganization. However, anecdotal evidence suggests that it is linked to greater empathy and compassion, higher levels of creativity and innovative thought, and the capacity to overcome fear-based blockages. These are just a few of the most profound and oft-cited results that have been described in the bulk of those who have used psilocybin.

As mentioned above, this is a subject that can be discussed extensively, and this book is dedicated more to safe use and psilocybin mushroom cultivation. However, before moving on, it is worthwhile to mention that moderate doses of psilocybin have been shown to shift the brain waves to the alpha rhythm, a state observed in both meditation and flow states. Higher doses have been linked to a dissolution of the ego, which, in turn, provides an opportunity to restructure our perception of ourselves and the world.

Microdosing

The use of psilocybin mushrooms and other psychedelics has historically been linked to powerful hallucinogenic experiences. Early research focused on the potential of psychedelics to induce mind-expanding spiritual experiences. These experiences were based on the capacity of large doses of psychedelic compounds to elicit profound changes in the perception of reality. However, in recent years, the practice of microdosing has been gaining attention. This involves the use of psychedelics to gain cognitive benefits without entering a full-blown trip.

Microdosing has, to some extent, increased the legitimacy of psychedelic use. One reason for this is that it is becoming popular among professionals in competitive industries such as those in Silicon Valley. By using a small amount of psilocybin or other psychedelic compounds, professionals are able to gain a competitive edge.

13

Microdosing can help a user to increase creativity and productivity while reducing the effects of anxiety and depression. Furthermore, this is a practice that can have lasting benefits, even after the regimen has been completed.

Essentially, microdosing is exactly what it sounds like. When on a psilocybin mushroom microdosing regimen, a user will ingest a small, measured dose of psilocybin mushrooms. The effect is sub-perceptual, meaning that it is below the amount needed for a psychedelic experience. After ingestion, the user will then go about work or their regular routine just as they would under normal circumstances.

Though the psychological effects are subtle, the benefits can still be profound. They include improved energy levels, problem-solving capacity, and focus. Anecdotal evidence also suggests that microdosing is helpful for breaking unhealthy habits and cultivating healthy ones, increasing connection with nature, improving diet, and improving relationships.

The process of microdosing psilocybin mushrooms is fairly simple. You'll want to begin with a batch of dried mushrooms. Psilocybin content can vary widely from one strain to the next and even from one mushroom to another in the same strain. Because of this, it is helpful to powder the entire batch and mix it together to equalize the levels of psilocybin throughout the batch. If you begin with fresh mushrooms, it will be helpful to boil a measured amount into a tea. Measure the weight of fresh mushrooms that go into the tea, and divide the volume of the resulting tea so that each dosage corresponds to 1g of the starting mass.

For most people, 0.1g of dried mushrooms or 1g of fresh mushrooms will be sufficient to gain the benefits of microdosing. You can use this as a starter dose and then adjust levels as necessary. The goal is to have enough so that you experience very little change in mood, mindset, or disposition, while still feeling extremely subtle effects. You may also need to "recalibrate" with each new batch. This is why it is helpful to have one of the microdosing days on the weekend. It's best to have a bit of a buffer in case the new batch is more potent than the previous. Most of the time, it's not all that fun to be full-on tripping at work.

Another key to microdosing is to set up a schedule. Tolerance will increase quickly, so it is ideal to give yourself two days between each dose. If you want to set up a weekly schedule, for example, you may wish to dose on Wednesday and Sunday. By dosing twice per week, you will gain the full benefits of microdosing without increasing tolerance and needing to up the dosage. Alternately, you can simply dose every three days. For example, dose on day 1, take days 2 and 3 off, then dose again on day 4.

Because microdosing is intended as a means of improving performance and generally enhancing life experience, it will help to keep a journal of the effects. You may wish to note the amount that you have ingested and any specific results you have noticed throughout the course of the day or week. Since psilocybin causes a reorganization of neural activity, it is helpful to record any observations during the off-days as well.

Plus, it is helpful to have records when experimenting with different dosages. You may wish to assess results in areas like productivity, creativity, anxiety, and focus. Different dosages will have different effects on each area, so keeping records will help you to find your "sweet spot" for different activities and effects.

When first beginning your microdosing regimen, you may wish to do so on a day off work. This will help you to become accustomed to the feeling and to make sure the dosage is right for you. You may wish to follow the regimen for several weeks to a few months at first, and then take some time off. In the process, you will be able to observe and record the short-term and long-term effects, and see how these effects persist after the regimen has been completed.

Remember that the goal is to integrate these benefits into your daily life without becoming dependent upon the psychedelic substance. With infrequent use, psilocybin can be leveraged as an occasional advantage. In addition, you'll find that the benefits will remain with you even when you are not actively ingesting psilocybin mushrooms. They essentially lead the way to productive mental and emotional states. This can help you to access these states without assistance in the future.

Finally, despite the numerous benefits of microdosing and of psychedelics in general, it is important to remember that these substances are not magical cure-alls. They can facilitate personal growth and healing, but it requires intention and focus to leverage these effects for lasting benefits. Plus, the key to the benefits provided by psilocybin and other psychedelics is awareness. Essentially, mindfulness. Psilocybin helps us to actively engage with our mental state. By becoming more aware of our internal states, our emotions, our thoughts, and our focus, we constructively harness our attention and access more of our natural potential.

Chapter 2

History of Psilocybin Mushrooms

The History

The psilocybin mushrooms have over two hundred varieties worldwide, each having slightly different effects and tastes. These mushrooms are commonly known as magic mushrooms, or shrooms, and are used as a recreational drug to induce hallucinations and an elated mood, the origins of which date back millennia.

Since it is nearly impossible to perfectly pinpoint the exact dates that the use of magic mushrooms became known, there is some evidence to indicate that aboriginal tribes from North Africa may have used psilocybin mushrooms since as early as 9000 BCE Rock paintings in Spain from around 6000 years ago also suggest that psilocybin mushrooms were used for religious rituals.

The possibility exists that the use of the mushroom even predates the Saharan aboriginal tribes, but we lack enough scientific evidence (Brusco, 2017).

The most widely known use of psilocybin mushrooms in history dates back to Native American cultures such as the Mayans and Aztecs, who used these mushrooms in many religious and spiritual rituals in order to communicate with their deific entities. However, there is a large gap between then and the time that Western civilization was introduced to psilocybin mushrooms.

It wasn't until the 1950s that author R. Gordon Wasson and French botanist Roger Heim identified the two compounds that gave the mushrooms their psychedelic quality, namely, psilocybin and psilocin.

Along with Albert Hoffman, they had collected samples from a Mazatec tribe during an expedition to Mexico, which Hoffman and Wasson had documented in their journals.

Shortly after the publication of a piece written by Wasson in Life magazine, the mushrooms gained popularity as a psychedelic substance which was hailed as the gateway to greater spiritualism.

Some archeological evidence from the desert explains and suggests that psychedelic mushrooms have been used by humans for a long time. Mushrooms are spoken of in prehistoric art across numerous different geographic locales. In most cases, they're thought to be strictly symbolic, often in the context of right of passage ceremonies. On the off chance that our precursors did use mushrooms, such a powerful experience almost positively would have influenced ancient culture, from art to religion to social values that directed everyday life.

Some have gone even further. Terence McKenna, for one, put forward the so-called "Stoned Ape Hypothesis," positing that early humans or pre-human primates ingested mushrooms, leading to evolutionary benefits including headways in intelligence. It ought to be noted that this speculation is respected with skepticism in the scientific community, considering some of McKenna's assumptions lack persuading evidence.

Even in pre-Columbian history, extensive and well-researched information has been obtained from the Aztec and Mayan societies of Mesoamerica, particularly in Mexico and Guatemala. After the vanquishing of these areas in the fifteenth and sixteenth hundreds of years, the Spanish restricted hallucinogenic mushroom use by indigenous peoples, regarding it as a barbaric and boorish cultural practice. Despite this, the indigenous shamans disregarded Spanish law in mystery for over 400 years to preserve their shared social legacy with these widely known mushrooms.

The first-ever known and reliable accounts in the western world of inebriation" with enchantment mushrooms came in 1799 when four children were accidentally fed Psilocybe semilanceata, a species of hallucinogenic mushroom.

The renowned Swiss scientific expert Albert Hofmann (who organized LSD) first segregated psilocybin in the lab in 1957 from Psilocybe Mexicana, a type of mushroom found fundamentally in Central America. After a year, it was created artificially just because. Gordon Wasson, previous unfortunate propensity leader of J. P. Morgan and Company, evidently had an intrigue that transformed into an obsession with psilocybin mushrooms. In 1955 he made an excursion to Oaxaca, Mexico, to meet Maria Sabina, an individual from the indigenous Mazatec Indian clan and a mushroom shaman. She exhibited Wasson to psilocybin mushrooms and spiritualist shamanism. On his first mushroom trip, he announced inclination "as though his spirit had been scooped out of his body."

Wasson effectively kick-started the hallucinogenic mushroom improvement in the West when, in 1957, Time Magazine appropriated his photograph paper titled "Looking for the Magic Mushroom," in which he itemized his encounters.

In the wake of scrutinizing of Wasson's experiences and after that heading out to Oaxaca to encounter psilocybin mushrooms for themselves, Timothy Leary and Richard Alpert, specialists at Harvard University, began the Harvard Psilocybin Project which, obviously, got them terminated immediately from that point. So they did what any jobless scholastic would have done in 1962: they began a hallucinogenic development. Psychedelic mushrooms were quickly embraced into the 1960s counterculture.

In 1971, psilocybin was recorded in the UN's Convention on Psychotropic Substances as a Schedule I sedate in the United States, making it illicit for all reasons. Regardless, psilocybin mushrooms were not part of the UN appear, which, right up 'til the present time, permits nations who have marked the show (basically a settlement) to control mushrooms that ordinarily contain psilocybin as they see fit. Today, psilocybin mushrooms are unlawful in most countries, even though there are exceptions.

Over the past few years, administrative bodies such as the DEA and FDA have loosened rules about utilizing psilocybin in controlled research trials more so than any other psychedelic. Energizing new research on psilocybin as both a therapeutic instrument and as a part of individual/otherworldly improvement strategies has been published and continues to be done today.

Psilocybin Mushrooms in Western Society

Western society has only encountered psychedelics relatively recently. This was largely due to Maria Sabina, a Mexican curandera, or native healer. Maria Sabina held healing rituals known as veladas. During these rituals, participants would ingest psilocybin mushrooms as a spiritual sacrament intended to purify and facilitate sacred communion. Sabina learned about the use of psilocybin mushrooms from her grandfather and great-grandfather, both shamans in the Mazatec tradition.

Valentina Wasson and R. Gordon Wasson were a married couple who were permitted by Maria Sabina to attend the velada in 1955. Their experience was so profound that they sought to make the potential of psilocybin mushrooms known to the West. Wasson collected spores from the mushrooms ingested during the ceremony. He brought these spores to Robert Heim, who, in the following year, identified them as members of the genus Psilocybe. Subsequent fieldwork allowed Heim to identify three species of Psilocybe used in the velada: Psilocybe mexicana, Psilocybe caerulescens, and Psilocybe zapotecorum. In 1957, the same year Albert Hoffman accidentally discovered LSD,

Wasson published an article in **Life** Magazine entitled "Seeking the Magic Mushroom." This made Wasson's experience available, at least in printed form, to the West. By 1958, Hoffman had identified psilocybin and psilocin as psychoactive compounds in psilocybin mushrooms. In the process, Hoffman began to synthesize psilocybin, making it possible for the purified compound to be tested in Western psychological trials.

Timothy Leary, after encountering Wasson's article, visited Mexico to gain firsthand experience of the psychedelic effects of psilocybin mushrooms. Leary returned to Harvard in 1960 and partnered with Richard Alpert to begin the Harvard Psilocybin Project. This project was a forum for the study of psychedelic substances, both from a psychological and spiritual standpoint. Though it led to the dismissal of Alpert and Leary from Harvard by 1963, their work and that of other contemporary researchers exploded into the popular field.

As Leary and Alpert continued to promote the psychedelic experience in 1960's counterculture, interest grew. As it did, both the use of psilocybin mushrooms and research into them expanded. By the beginning of the next decade, several Psilocybe species had been identified throughout North America, Asia, and Europe. As these mushrooms are naturally occurring across the world, positive identification was followed by collection. During this period, a number of works were also published detailing how to cultivate Psilocybe cubensis. P. cubensis is a species of psilocybin mushroom which is extremely hardy and relatively easy to grow. This makes it a perfect specimen for cultivation by novices with limited materials.

In the present day, psilocybin mushrooms are among the most widely-used psychedelic substances. They are readily available in nature and easy to cultivate. Furthermore, they have been described in the 2017 Global Drug Survey as the safest recreational drug. Despite this, the active compounds of psilocybin mushrooms, psilocybin, and psilocin were declared in 1968 to be as illegal in their purified form as heroin and crack cocaine. Legality of the mushrooms themselves varies by country and will be discussed in greater detail in later sections.

Current usage

Psilocybin mushrooms are the most generally utilized psychedelics among people ages 34 and below.

A recent report of 409 university students in the American northeast discovered that almost 30% of those surveyed had attempted psilocybin magic mushrooms not less than three times.

Surveys in 12 EU parts discovered that people aged 15–24 years old use of enchantment mushrooms ranges from under 1% to 8%

In the UK, almost 340,000 people aged 16–59 had used enchantment mushrooms in the most recent year as of 2004/2005, right before they were made completely illegal in the UK.

Early Use of Psilocybin

Though we don't know when humans first discovered psychoactive mushrooms, archeological findings suggest that they have been known and used by early human tribes at least 9000 years ago. Some of the earliest evidence comes from stone-age art. Depictions of mushrooms can be found in cave paintings discovered near Villa del Homo, Spain and in the Tassili caves in southern Algeria. These have led archeologists to hypothesize that early humans used psychedelic mushrooms in religious rituals.

One theory, posited by Terrence McKenna, is that psychedelic mushrooms were a central influence in human evolution. McKenna has posited that magic mushrooms helped to raise human consciousness to the level of self-reflection and abstract thought. This theory has been criticized by the scientific community as being lacking in evidence. However, current studies into the impact of psychedelics on brain function suggest that they have the capacity to reorganize neural connections and increase communication between different parts of the brain. To me, this suggests that there might be more to McKenna's theory than the scientific community has yet recognized.

To bring this to (relatively) more modern times, numerous stone carvings depicting mushrooms have been found in Central and South America. Many of these statues and murals date back more than 2000 years and have marked similarity to specific Psilocybe species. The Mayan, Aztec, Mazatec, Nahua, Mixtec, and Zapotec tribes of Central America are all known to have used psychedelic mushrooms in their religious rituals. The Aztecs called one Psilocybe species teonanacatl, meaning "flesh of the gods." Mazatec and Aztec names for psilocybin mushrooms can be translated to "wondrous mushrooms," "divinatory mushrooms," and "genius mushrooms."

The use of psilocybin mushrooms was prevalent amongst these tribes when the Spanish conquistadors arrived in the New World. However, the Spanish viewed their use with suspicion, believing that they allowed users to communicate with devils. Therefore, the use of Psilocybes and other psychedelic substances was suppressed. Efforts to convert the tribes to Catholicism also resulted in the suppression of all religious and spiritual traditions of the tribes. However, tribal religious practices, including those which use entheogens (psychedelic substances), have persisted, often in secret, into the present day.

Chapter 3

Medical uses of Psilocybin Mushrooms

Mushrooms for Cancer Treatment

These days, mushrooms are all about the excitement of complementary and free cancer treatments. It seems unlikely. Mushrooms can be slimy, poisonous, and fungal to the right. However, science takes a serious look at medicinal mushrooms and how they fight cancer, tumors, syndrome of chronic fatigue, and autoimmune diseases. Every day, further studies show that medicinal mushrooms improve resistance, fight cancer, and reduce tumors. If you're looking for cancer treatment mushrooms, this book will give you a brief overview of mushrooms from around the world that have proven their effectiveness in fighting cancer.

Science is proving what Eastern Medicine has known for centuries in the research on medicinal mushrooms. Mushrooms have been commonly used for thousands of years in China and Japan. Mushrooms including Reishi, Shiitake, Maitake, and Lion's Mane are used by traditional Chinese medicine doctors to encourage durability and keep body systems healthy and strong. Mushrooms promote "chi" flow throughout the body, increase energy, remove toxins, and create an overall sense of well-being. In the fight against cancer, medicine takes a serious dig at mushrooms. More studies on the anti-cancer effects of wild mushrooms are being carried out. Wild mushroom compounds are used to treat cancer in many parts of the world.

The Reishi, also known as Ganoderma lucidum, is one of the most famous medicinal mushrooms. This fungus is classified as "The Immortality Fungus" and has been used in Eastern Medicine for at least 3000 years. Reishi mushroom was officially listed as an alternative herb for cancer treatment by the Japanese government in 1990. Reishi is used in cancer research centers around the world with favorable results. Reishi may be one of the most well-known and widely used medicinal mushrooms in the world. It is distributed in the whole shape, a dense shelf fungus, as well as in the form of tincture, paste and tablets.

Chaga, also known as Inonotus obliquus, is used for the treatment of cancer around the globe. Historically, the mushroom has been used by Russian legends in Poland and Western Siberia for decades, speaking of a fungus which develops on birch trees that are effective in treating a number of cancers. Chaga "tea" is a mushroom infusion given to patients with cancer. The U.S. National Cancer Institute reported using Chaga to treat cancer effectively. Chaga appears to be one of the most effective cancer treatment medicinal mushrooms.

Tramates versicolor, commonly known as the Turkey Tail fungus, is one of the most widely available fungi for cancer treatment. This spreads prolifically throughout North America and is used to fight cancer widely around the globe. PSK, known as the "Kureha polysaccharide," is a Turkey Tail mushroom type. Through scientific studies, through conjunction with radiation and chemotherapy, PSK's anti-tumor function is improved. Improved survival rates are widespread in patients taking PSK. In one study, the cancer death rate was 21% with PSK and 52% without within 5 years.

The Reishi, Chaga, and Turkey Tail are three big cancer mushrooms from around the globe. All of these are available online and in local food stores.

Healing with herbs, particularly in cancer treatment, is becoming more common as an adjunct therapy; but what about mushroom healing? Herbs are called food for crops. Where does the mushroom fit? Herbs are herbaceous plants from a botanical point of view. Herbal medicine may use leaves, roots, and flowers. The kingdom of plants is made up of plants. The world of fungi is made up of mushrooms. Research is investigating the importance of medicinal mushrooms in the diagnosis of severe medical problems, including autoimmune disease, nervous disorders and cancer. This book reveals some of the mystery surrounding mushrooms and looks at their use in natural medicine for a short time.

Many legends accompany the Kingdom Fungi. "Well, some mushrooms are poisonous," you might think. And yes, that's true. Many crops are poisonous as well. Mushrooms get a bad reputation because they often attract a lot of attention in cases of mushroom poisoning. Most of the mushrooms are not poisonous. You might think, "Will I see visions or hallucinate?" Many cultures around the world use hallucinogenic healing mushrooms. But in labs around the globe, medicinal mushrooms are being studied, and physicians, cancer specialists, and alternative medicine practitioners are treating mushrooms seriously and recommending them for severe medical conditions.

What are the medicinal mushrooms? Check first at the polypore, or shelf fungi, while looking for mushrooms to cure cancer. From an evolutionary point of view, these fungi are the youngest. Most mycologists (those researching fungi) assume that polypore have formed from all the mushrooms. Polypores are as hard as gilled spores, not as soft. It must first be cooked, heated, or tenderized for any mushroom to be digestible. In the case of polypore mushrooms this is particularly true. Next, they need to be warmed to be usable organically. Historically, polypore mushrooms are roasted and steeped in hot water, filtered and eaten as a mushroom tea for the subsequent beverage.

Historically, polypore mushrooms have been of great value to the world's indigenous peoples. Many rough, shelf mushrooms have been used as tinder or spunk for starting fires and going on long distances. These same plants have also been sliced and steeped for tea in rain. On every world, shamans of communities handled severe medical problems with polypore mushrooms.

Which mushrooms are polypore mushrooms for cancer treatment? The Reishi mushroom is the most popular and widely used polypore mushroom. It is commonly used by traditional Japanese practitioners in Traditional Chinese Medicine, and throughout China, Vietnam, and Eastern cultures. The medicinal mushroom, also known as the Ling Chi, is available online and directly from traditional medical practitioners in additional shape.

Grifola frondosa, also known as Maitake, is another important medicinal polypore mushroom. Maitake is a nutritionally and medicinally valued soft fleshed polypore. It attracts a lot of interest from pharmaceutical and neutraceutical firms since initial studies indicate that as an anti-tumor drug it is quite active, especially in cases of liver and breast cancer. Search for nutrients from Maitake which deal with D-fraction and beta-glucans. Maitake drugs are widely available from organic clinics and on the internet.

It makes sense that the mysterious fungi hold healing power after dissolving some of the myths around mushrooms and exploring the history of mushrooms as medicine briefly.

Button Mushroom and Cardiovascular Disease (CVD)

Strong evidence from epidemiological studies suggests that regular fruit and vegetable consumption is strongly associated with reduced cardiovascular disease (CVD) risk. Dietary mushrooms, for instance, can defend against chronic disease by modifying inflammatory environments and inhibiting cellular processes under pro-inflammatory conditions correlated with CVD.

These findings have been shown to support the notion of dietary mushrooms in CVD protection, but multi canters and large sample size studies are needed to identify the main ingredient that is comparable to the current medicine used to enhance its validation.

Nonetheless, the University of Gdansk report in reviews and updates evidence on macro and trace elements and Radionuclides in edible wild-grown and cultivated mushrooms indicated that the coexistence of minerals with nutritional value obtained from natural habitats and co-occurrence with some harmful elements like Cd, Pb, Hg, Ag, As, and Radionuclides should be taken with certain precautions.

Medicinal Mushrooms in Effective Treatment of Erectile Dysfunction-Impotence and Low Libido

Their cellular components can have a profound impact on human health quality. These health and healing agents, even at high doses, are extremely low in toxicity. For most pharmaceutical drugs, this is not the case.

Mushrooms have been widely used in China's royal palaces. Cordyceps was the option of fungus. Historically, its use was limited to the emperors and their concubines exclusively.

Cordyceps research done at the Beijing Medical University in China, as well as in Japan, found a 64 percent success rate in people with impotence relative with 24 percent in the placebo group.

Cordyceps are extremely expensive as they grow normally in the wild. It's a host's fungal development and worms its way into the hosting skin. This may sound horrific, but not only does the drug work but it performs very well.

Today, a Cordyceps has been developed by science and technology that does not feed on a host and is grown according to organic standards. It makes the Cordyceps raised vegetarian.

There are many curative medicinal mushrooms, and these are described below. Remember that the Cordyceps are the best overall mushroom to carry.

Sexual Potentiator: Cordyceps (Cordyceps sinesis); Shiitake / Xiang Gu (Lentinula edodes) Libido Tonic: Cordyceps (Cordyceps sinesis); Shiitake / Xiang Gu (Lentinula edodes); Reishi / Ling Zhi (Ganoderma lucidum); Turkish Tail / Yun Zhi (Trametes versicolor) Regulate Blood Pressure: Cordyceps (Cordyceps sinesis); Shiitake / Xiang Gu (Lentinula edodes); Reishi / Ling Zhi (Ganoderma lucidum); Get mushrooms to crack and dose. And don't overlook that if you're able to fork out the cash, the Cordyceps is the best overall mushroom. The best choice could be the natural vegetarian one!

Mushrooms Are Valuable Food— Increasing Oxygen Efficiency and Disease Resistance With advances in refrigeration and transportation technology and new cultivation methods being adopted, mushrooms are now being sold in grocery stores along with apples, squash and pumpkins. You will now get a wide variety of mushrooms that just a few years ago would have been impossible.

Mushrooms have always attracted people to their different shapes, sizes and textures. If they don't cook, people want to know what they are and how they can be made.

The value of eating mushrooms is only recently recognized by Americans, a fact that has been acknowledged to other peoples for decades. Mushrooms have low calories, but high protein content. They also contain zinc, iron, chitin, minerals, vitamins and dietary fibers that make them a healthy option.

Mushrooms are also widely used to prepare alternative medicines in addition to being healthy food items. Mushrooms have been used in traditional Chinese medicine (TCM) for hundreds of years. More than 200 mushroom species are present in China and about 25% of them have anti-carcinogenic properties.

Mushrooms are also an origin of germanium, and a substance believed to improve the body's oxygen production. It is also known that germanium balances the amount of exposure the body has to pollutants from the environment and helps boost the body's immunity. Germanium is also known to neutralize the remains of toxins in the body in addition to these beneficial effects.

The Shiitake, Reishi and Maitake are the three most popular medicinal mushrooms. If you get a chance, these mushrooms should be eaten at least once a week.

Everywhere from hospitals to pharmacy and supermarkets, Love Mushrooms to Avoid Flu vaccines are sold. While the Centers for Disease Control and Prevention states that the flu vaccine's main side effects include redness, soreness, and swelling at the shot location, low-grade cough, and aches, some suggest the vaccines contain mercury and other issue ingredients and are more dangerous than the flu itself.

In addition, there are literally thousands of strains of the flu virus, but only a few are selected and targeted by the vaccines marketed each year, which health officials believe will be the most prevalent of the flu season. They often don't think they're right.

But there were flu-fighting fungi even before there were effective vaccinations. For thousands of years, the Chinese have used mushrooms as medicine, and recent scientific findings have indicated that mushrooms are active in improving the immune system. So the best defense against flu is a good immune system right now.

The world's most popular grown edible mushroom is the mushroom button that was believed to have no nutritious or therapeutic quality for many years. Nevertheless, recent studies have shown that the lowly key, as well as crimini and portobello, have as much antioxidant capacity as their Asian equivalents, which have been admired for their disease prevention and healing properties for generations. Among other compounds that stimulate the immune system and serve as free radical scavengers, buttons in particular include polysaccharides and ergothioneine.

Shiitake and Maitake mushrooms in Japanese medicine, now widely available on U.S. markets, have been so effective in improving the immune system and fighting cancer that they are now being screened for HIV. Enoki mushrooms have also proven benefits for the immune system.

Chinese medicine is also a staple of Reishi mushrooms. These are found in teas, extracts and tablets, although they are not nutritious, and are used to enhance immunity and reduce inflammation.

Mushrooms are a good source of B vitamins like niacin, which contain the enzymes required to turn carbohydrates into fuel, and riboflavin, which converts certain nutrients such as vitamin B6 and folate into functional forms.

Champignons are fat-free, high in fiber and calcium, and a strong potassium origin. These are flexible and simple to integrate in your daily diet, most significantly. All it takes to get the benefits is a one-half cup. Apply in soups, stews, grains and vegetables, or add them in your salad.

Apply a number of mushrooms to your meals today and every day to combat the flu or any other pandemic you're living through.

Chapter 4

What is a Magic Mushroom

Magic mushrooms, as they're understood, are naturally occurring fungi that are ordinarily consumed raw or dried and can be consumed in coffee or tea. These mushrooms create hallucinogenic effects on the consumer.

Undoubtedly, the food eaten in the natural season and grown on-site tastes much better. Mushrooms are in season; there are a number of fine recipes, including delicious and versatile mushrooms. If you set off near a green, the temptation is to commit this cute little vegetable with a warning: Know your mushrooms before you cook them. Rarely, these are the ones that kill dinner, but they can really make people sick. There is another consideration, though it is great fun to pick your own food with mushrooms; they are very cumbersome and require a lot of rinsing before you can get rid of all the dirt. If you have decided to pick instead of the supermarket, use a knife to cut the mushroom clean and do not pull it. Take, for example, the chanterelles, these beautiful mushrooms have an exquisite consistency and are probably the most versatile of all wild mushrooms, as they have so many uses in cooking. Excellent for preparing recipes with fish, the perfect partner for game, beef, and duck, as in the best restaurants. All cooks who are often versed in dieting will explain the mushroom's magic through little-known simple facts:

Mushrooms contain the triple antioxidant than tomatoes -14 mushrooms or 80g serving count for the goal of 5 A DAY - They are a good source of easily absorbable high-quality protein that contains more than other vegetable Mushrooms are low in carbohydrates and fat. Magic mushrooms have a very positive effect on our health. Mushrooms are rich in phytochemicals to fight diseases. If you eat mushrooms regularly, there is a lower risk of breast cancer. Fungi also prevent the proliferation of prostate cancer cells. They provide hard-to-get nutrients. A medium-sized mushroom offers 21 percent of the recommended daily intake of selenium and one-third of your copper requirement. Oyster mushrooms are an excellent source of iron. Mushrooms retain their nutrients when roasted, grilled, or cooked in the microwave, and can help cut kilojoules. When mushrooms replaced minced meat in dishes such as lasagna and chili con carne, adults consumed 1600 kilojoules less per day. Mushrooms relieve cardiovascular disease by lowering blood pressure and cholesterol. They also help to reduce insulin resistance, which increases insulin sensitivity and blocks the growth of cancerous tumors. They strengthen our immune system and reduce the toxic levels of the estrogen hormone. They are anti-inflammatory, and they have strong antioxidant properties. They reduce the hormone-dependent breast cancer. They have analgesic, anti-inflammatory properties. They help combat infections, increase libido, and also combat allergies.

A medium-sized Portabella mushroom has even more potassium than a banana or a glass of orange juice. A serving of mushrooms also provides about 20 to 40 percent of the daily value of copper, a mineral with cardio-protective properties.

They contain about 80 to 90 percent of water and are very low in calories. They have little sodium and fat, and 8 to 10 percent of dry weight is fiber. Therefore, they are an ideal food for people undergoing a weight management program. They have a type of carbohydrate that helps to stabilize blood sugar while keeping your metabolism high. Consuming 3 ounces of mushrooms a day helps you burn more calories and lose up to 13 pounds in five weeks, according to study. Natural compound in shiitakes, known as lentinan, invigorates white blood cells to fight off infections. Gandodermic acid, a drug of Reishis, helps control cholesterol levels by 12%, helps to reduce the plaque that causes clogged arteries by 2/3, and can lower blood pressure by 12%. If you eat just a few ounces a day, relax and keep the arteries free. Mushrooms naturally contain vitamin D. They are the only non-animal foods that contain natural vitamin D, which is automatically produced when exposed to light. They contain beta-glucans, which can protect against certain types of cancer, such as breast, skin, stomach, and lung cancer. It has been shown that beta-glucans in fungi can transport immune cells into the cancerous area and destroy cancer cells. Who would have thought that some kinds of mushrooms have magical health benefits? Breast cancer is the most common cancer among women worldwide and that its rate is rising in both developed and developing countries.

Interestingly, the cancer incidence in China was four to five times lower than in industrialized countries. The use of dried and fresh mushrooms and green leaf tea in the traditional Chinese diet. Mushrooms extracts and green tea showed carcinogenic properties that were thought to stimulate the immune response. The consumption of mushrooms and green tea by 2,000 women aged 20 to 87 years in relatively prosperous southeast China was monitored.

The results of the study showed that combining fungal and green tea intake reduced the risk of breast cancer and further reduced the malignancy of cancer. The Agaricusblazei fungus is composed of beta- (1-3) -D-glucan, beta- (1-4) -a-D-glucan and beta - (1-6) -D-glucan. These immune-enhancing substances known as beta-glucan have been shown to have very strong anti-tumor properties. While they do not directly damage the anti-tumor effect, they trigger the body's own anti-tumor reaction. One type of anti-tumor leukocyte, known as natural killer (NK) cells, is produced by the body, which makes it relatively easy to measure the level of NK cells in the body. When Agari is administered to human subjects in their diet, a 300% increase in NK cells in the blood is observed within 2 to 4 days. The natural killer cells are best known for their ability to kill tumor cells before they develop into cancer. However, there are also indications of their role in controlling infections in the early stages of the body's immune response.

The Piedade mushroom found in the rainforests is internationally known for its healing properties. After several clinical trials, the Piedade fungus and the Agaricusblazei fungus cultured in the mountainous region of California were combined to form a super-hybrid and effective fungal fluid. This product uses a 10-step extraction technology that captures all nutritious elements and, a powerful antioxidant, is considered to be a powerhouse of nutrients essential for maintaining a healthy and active lifestyle, We no longer have to go to the rainforest in Brazil or scale the mountains in California to find this pure gold.

According to researchers, magic mushrooms relieve anxiety and depression, because they feel affectionate and are "one" with everything. This leads to a change in the brain or neuroplasticity. "Studies in MRI imaging show that psilocybin alters brain activity and allows communication between regions of your brain that normally do not connect, which is considered part of the breakthroughs reported by humans." The benefits of magic mushrooms seem promising, "When someone goes out and does it themselves, they can feel tremendous fear and paranoia and feel much worse. Even in controlled situations, we are still very worried about the result of magic mushrooms. This reminds us of how most people claim that marijuana bong hits have few or no side effects.

Instead of masking depression and anxiety with medications and suffering from the side effects, how about identifying the cause of the problem and how to deal with it? We noticed that most problems have a physical, emotional, mental, and spiritual effect. Sometimes, when you address the spiritual effects, the others are easier to treat or even disappear.

When we feel anxiety or depression, we spend 10 minutes reading the script aloud. In this way, we summon powerful spiritual helpers from the other side to eliminate the invisible garbage, and we immediately feel better. It's so easy that some people have a hard time believing it until they try it and see the results.

Just as everyone is physically polluted by daily life, everyone takes in negative energy everywhere, sometimes in the form of ginned and dark entities. The more empathetic and sensitive you are, the more you would benefit from regular clearing. Dietary changes and regular exercise are more effective than depression medications.

Magic mushrooms, as they are called, are naturally occurring mushrooms that are normally eaten raw or dried and ground and drunk in tea or coffee, producing hallucinogenic effects.

This can be an irresistible enticement to the thrill-seeking mushroom user, who collects it at their own discretion as each mushroom is intended for consumption. However, not all of these fungi are desired, and it can be very difficult to distinguish those that are toxic or not. Some of these fungi are highly toxic and can kill very slowly and painfully, such as fever, vomiting, and diarrhea. Some even have a delayed reaction that takes days to show any signs or symptoms before taking your life without an antivenin.

Since Magic Mushrooms are found in nature and in no way "processed" before consumption, they are considered a safe drug. Absolutely no drug is safe, and most drugs are naturally occurring or, in any case, refined from natural plants or fungi. However, they are neither known as addictive substances or heavy drugs nor as violent or psychologically harmful as LSD or as socially corrosive substances such as crackers or heroin. However, depending on the mental disposition of the fungal user, fungi can have deleterious effects on the user. For example, if the user is prone to a fragile mental state or is very suggestible in nature, he may believe that his hallucinations are the manifestation of something true, and some of it is possessed and thereby damaged. One such documented case of these extremities involved a young man who began to take mushrooms and have the recurrent hallucination of a flower disguised as a court jester, repeatedly insulting him with scars. As absurd as it sounds, without any of these experiences as hallucinations, he believed that this abusive flower was the manifestation of truths about itself and turned into a major depression. He and his friends admitted that he was fine before picking mushrooms, but at some point during the course, he opened a can of worms. Unfortunately, he still struggles with emotional and mental issues that were simply not there before the onset of his life-changing hallucinations. In such a case, one can not say with certainty whether the fungi were responsible for triggering such persistent psychological problems, or whether there was already an underlying mental illness and the fungus use was insignificant, but it is always to be considered.

Chapter 5

Different types of Magic Mushrooms

Edible mushrooms

Many of the more than 2,500 domestic mushroom species are edible - but far from all. The following overview presents the 30 most popular mushrooms in alphabetical order with their characteristic properties, classic locations and harvest time. If available, the list draws attention to the distinguishing features of toxic counterparts.

Birch mushroom (Leccinum scabrum)

Habit: 5 to 15 cm high, hemispherical, later flattened hat, 5 to 15 cm tall

Hat color: light gray-brown with reddish shimmer or yellowish nuances

Handle color: white, often with black net or black scales, similar to a birch trunk

Tubes (sponge): white on young mushrooms, later ocher yellow

Occurrence: in symbiosis under birch trees

Collection time: June to November

Flavor: mild to sour

Risk of confusion: unmistakable thanks to the characteristic handle

Bratling (Lactarius volemus)

Growth habit: 10 to 12 cm high, 5 to 15 cm wide, flat hat with dent in the middle

Hat color: orange-red-brown to cinnamon, rarely bread yellow

Handle color: orange-brown

Slats: yellow with red discoloration at pressure points

Occurrence: on the edges of deciduous and coniferous forests

Collection time: July to October

Flavor: mild

Risk of confusion: unmistakable thanks to the pungent fish smell of herring

Special feature: strong milk flow occurs even with small injuries and turns the fingers brown

Bronze boletus, black-capped boletus (Boletus aereus)

Growth habit: 15 cm high, 3 to 5 cm thick stem, hemispherical, up to 25 cm tall hat, velvety skin

Hat color: black to ocher-brown

Handle color: creamy yellow to creamy white

Tubes (sponge): white

Occurrence: under chestnuts and oaks

Collection time: July to October

Flavor: nutty and mild

Risk of confusion: none, resembles other boletus mushrooms, all of which are edible

Special feature: mushroom of the year 2008, one of the most impressive, edible mushrooms on home soil

Thin meat anise mushroom (Agaricus silvicola)

Form of growth: 8 to 10 cm high, thin hat with 5 to 10 cm diameter, first bell-shaped, later flat screened

Hat color: sulfur yellow to cream with yellow spots

Stem: white, hollow inside, slim, 1 to 1.5 cm thick, bulbous foot

Slats: pink, brown with age

Occurrence: deciduous and coniferous forests

Collection time: June to October

Risk of confusion: poisonous tuberous agaric with white lamellae

Special feature: intense scent of anise or almonds

Noble stimulus, blood stimulus (Lactarius deliciosus)

Growth habit: 3 to 7 cm high, 5 to 10 cm wide, with a hollow foot when old

Hat: first flat, later funnel-shaped to rolled up, brick-orange with shades, silvery stripes

Handle color: orange

Slats: ocher yellow to light orange

Occurrence: pine forests

Collection time: August to October

Flavor: mild, fruity

Risk of confusion: irritant salmon, which is not poisonous but has an extremely bitter taste

Special feature: orange milk turns the urine red after consumption, which is harmless

Bottle Dustling (Lycoperdon perlatum)

Growth habit: prickly, white shape, 3 to 10 cm tall, no pronounced hat

Handle color: white for young mushrooms, brown for older specimens

Occurrence: coniferous forests, rarely in deciduous forests

Collection time: June to October

Risk of confusion: poisonous potato biscuit with yellow-brown warts and black meat inside

Special feature: brown meat from older mushrooms is inedible

Female pigeon (Russula cyanoxantha)

Habit: 5 to 15 cm wide, flat hat

Hat color: violet-green, more rarely ocher-yellow

Stem: 4 to 10 cm high, 1 to 4 cm thick, whitish with a purple hue

Slats: white

Occurrence: beech forests and in mixed forests

Collection time: July to October

Flavor: pleasantly mild

Risk of confusion: with other pigeons whose bitter taste can numb the tongue

Special feature: mushroom of the year 1997

European Boletus (Suillus grevillei)

Growth habit: first hemispherical, later flat hat, 5 to 15 cm wide

Hat color: gold-yellow to orange-brown

Stem: yellowish, 4 to 10 cm high and 0.5 to 2 cm wide, white skin ring

Tubes (sponge): yellowish, brown when old

Occurrence: among larches in symbiotic community

Collection time: July to October

Flavor: spicy-mild, with tender meat

Risk of confusion: none

Hawk mushroom, venison mushroom (Sarcodon imbricatus)

Habit: 5 to 8 cm high with a hat up to 15 cm wide, spiky underneath

Hat: scaly and light brown like the plumage of hawk and sparrow hawk, with a sunken middle

Stem: 2 to 5 cm wide, initially white, later turns brown from the base

Slats: light gray, spiky

Occurrence: in beech and spruce forests, often in closed witch rings

Collection time: June to November

Flavor: mild to nutty-spicy

Danger of confusion: due to the spiky underside of the hat, easy to identify even by laypersons

Special feature: mushroom of the year 1996

Hornbeam bolete (Leccinum carpini)

Growth habit: wrinkled hat with a diameter of up to 12 cm

Hat color: light brown to dark brown

Handle color: greyish with dark scales

Tubes: bulge-like bulge around the stem gray-white, later gray-green

Occurrence: among hornbeams and hornbeam hedges

Collection time: July to October

Flavor: pleasantly mild

Risk of confusion: none, resembles the edible birch mushroom

Special feature: after being cut, the meat turns purple to black, which does not affect the taste

Fall Trumpet (Craterellus cornucopioides)

Growth habit: funnel-shaped, hollow fruiting body, 2 to 6 cm wide, 3 to 12 cm tall

Hat color: black inside, brown-black outside with folded edge

Handle color: gray

Occurrence: mainly under beech trees, otherwise in beech and fir forests

Collection time: August to November

Flavor: mild

Danger of confusion: Gray performance with 1-6 cm wide, gray-brown funnel hat

Judas ear (Auricularia)

Form of growth: 4 to 10 cm wide, elastic fruiting body reminds of an auricle

Fruit body color: reddish brown, olive brown to greyish violet

Flesh color: reddish brown

Occurrence: mainly on the wood of the black elder and on other deciduous trees

Collection time: all year round

Flavor: very mild

Risk of confusion: unmistakable due to the bizarre shape

Special feature: Mushroom of the year 2017, contracts when it is dry and swells when it is wet

Curled hen, curled hen (Sparassis crispa)

Growth habit: frizzy fruiting bodies, 10 to 40 cm in diameter, resembles a bath sponge

Color fruiting body: yellowish to light brown

Flesh color: white-yellow

Stalk: thick fleshy base, reminiscent of a cauliflower drink

Occurrence: pines

Collection time: July to November

Taste: very tasty, mild nutty, the lighter the flesh, the more delicate

Risk of confusion: none, the similar looking oak hen is also edible

May mushroom (Calocybe gambosa)

Habit: 5 to 8 cm high, 3 to 10 cm wide, initially closed, later spread hat, rolled up edge

Hat color: cream-white

Handle color: cream-white

Slats: cream-white

Occurrence: on forest edges

Collection time: May and June

Flavor: mild

Risk of confusion: highly toxic brick-red crack fungus, optical double, whose fruit-like scent serves as the most important distinguishing feature

Special feature: more intense, than obtrusive, mealy smell that disappears when cooking

Chestnut Boletus (Xerocomus badius)

Growth habit: 12 cm high, 3 cm wide, semicircular

Hat color: brownish, matt, greasy when wet

Handle color: yellow-brown

Tubes (sponge): cream-yellow, discolored bluish with slight pressure

Occurrence: Spruce and pine forests

Collection time: June to November

Flavor: nutty, mildly aromatic

Risk of confusion with toadstools: none

Black-headed milkling (Lactarius lignyotus)

Growth habit: hat with rolled edge, 2 to 6 cm wide, grooved stem

Hat color: black-brown to soot-colored

Handle color: black-brown

Flesh color: white

Slats: white

Occurrence: spruce forests

Collection time: August to October

Taste: mild, but the milk can taste bitter

Risk of confusion: pitch-black milkling, unground, darker stem, hunched over, causes stomach upset

Monk's head (Clitocybe geotropa)

Form of growth: 8 to 15 cm tall, with up to 25 cm wide, spreading hat and wart-like hump

Hat color: cream to beige, brownish in age

Handle color: cream to beige

Slats: white to off-white, down the stem

Occurrence: deciduous and coniferous forests

Collection time: September to November

Risk of confusion: highly poisonous white varnished funnel, only half the size and with no hump on the hat

Special feature: gathers up to 800 m tall witch rings

Pearl mushroom (Amanita rubescens)

Growth habit: spherical, later screened hat, up to 15 cm tall

Hat color: light brown, set with pink-gray pearl flakes

Handle color: white with a reddish tinge, fluted ring

Slats: white, spotted pink when aged

Occurrence: deciduous and coniferous forests

Collection time: June to October

Taste: mild, sweet, raw poisonous

Danger of confusion: panther mushroom, very poisonous, white stem without red shimmer, hat with smaller pearl flakes

Special feature: the pearl-like flakes disappear from the hat when it rains

Chanterelle (Cantharellus cibarius)

Growth habit: hemispherical, short-stemmed, 3 to 8 cm tall

Hat: bright yellow, 3 to 12 cm in size, changing shapes from deep recessed to arched to funnel-shaped

Stem: thin, grooved and yellow

Slats: yellowish and forked

Occurrence: coniferous forests, mainly in nests under pines

Collection time: June to October

Flavor: spicy to slightly peppery

Risk of confusion: none, resembles the false chanterelle, which tastes bland

Special feature: is under nature protection and may only be collected for personal use

Giant umbrella (Macrolepiota procera)

Growth habit: 15 to 40 cm high, young hat round, screened up to 40 cm tall, with a slight hump in the middle

Hat color: cream-colored with dark scales

Handle: slim, hollow, with a sliding ring, gray-brown

Slats: creamy white, later brownish

Occurrence: in clearings and on the edges of deciduous forests, in parks and in cemeteries

Collection time: June to November

Taste: nutty to mild, especially the ring

Risk of confusion: poison saffron umbrella, 5 to 30 cm tall, light-colored hat with dark spots, causes stomach upset

Special feature: edible mushroom of the year in 2017, still raw poisonous

Sheep champignon (Agaricus arvensis)

Habit: 5 to 15 cm high, hemispherical to slightly arched, very meaty hat, up to 15 cm in diameter

Hat color: cream-colored, smooth surface

Handle color: cream to dirty yellow

Slats: gray-white to pink and brownish

Occurrence: meadows, parks, pastures

Collection time: May to October

Flavor: tasty, mildly pleasant

Danger of confusion: highly toxic carbol mushroom, very similar in appearance, carbol-like, unpleasant smell is the most important distinguishing feature; deadly poisonous spring tuber agaric, recognizable by pure white lamellae, therefore please exercise extreme caution with young mushrooms that still thrive with white lamellae

Crested Inkling (Coprinus comatus)

Growth habit: 10 to 25 cm high with a cylindrical hat

Hat: 5 to 10 cm high, 3 to 6 cm wide, white with brown scales

Handle color: white

Slats: white

Occurrence: rubble sites, fields and roadsides, meadows, rarely in forests

Collection time: May to November

Taste: mild, delicate, but only with young mushrooms

Risk of confusion: unmistakable

Special feature: old specimens melt away, like dark ink

Pig's ear, purple cuckoo (Gomphus clavatus)

Growth habit: 2 to 8 cm high, 4 to 8 cm wide, often intertwined, funnel-shaped fruiting bodies, wavy edge

Fruit color: flesh-colored to purple

Last on the outside: flesh-colored, longitudinally veined, forked

Occurrence: beech and spruce forests

Collection time: August to October

Danger of confusion: due to the unusual shape, unmistakable even for laypeople

Special feature: mushroom of the year 1998, is under nature protection, collecting for own use is allowed

Food morel (Morchella esculenta)

Growth habit: 10 to 30 cm in size, oval to egg-shaped with round, honeycomb-shaped ribs

Hat color: light beige to brownish

Handle color: white, lighter than the hat

Occurrence: deciduous forests, parks

Collection time: April to May

Danger of confusion: none, resembles the less tasty pointed morels with a pointed, net-like hat

Special feature: is under nature protection, collecting for personal use is allowed

Boletus, spruce boletus, male mushroom (Boletus edulis)

Growth habit: thick tube, rounded, domed hat

Hat color: brown

Stem: pale brown, thick-bellied, barrel to roller-shaped, with a light mesh pattern

Tubes (sponge): with increasing age from white to yellowish to green

Occurrence: coniferous and deciduous forests

Collection time: June to October

Flavor: nutty

Danger of confusion: none, resembles non-toxic, bitter, light brown gall blanks with a pink underside

Special feature: is under nature protection, picking for own use is allowed

Stick sponges (Kuehneromyces mutabilis)

Growth habit: 5 cm high, 4 cm wide,

Hat color: brown, damp shiny

Stem: a ring separates the smooth, upper, cream-colored half from the scaly, dark, lower half of the stalk

Slats: cream white

Occurrence: deciduous forests

Collection time: April to November

Flavor: spicy

Danger of confusion: poison-dove with a smooth, cream-colored to brown stem as the only distinguishing feature

Violet lacquer funnel (Laccaria amethystina)

Habit: 4 to 10 cm high, 2 to 6 cm tall, flat to domed hat

Hat color: when wet: intense violet, the drier the paler

Handle color: violet, fibrous

Slats: purple, strikingly far apart

Occurrence: deciduous and fir forests and in parks

Collection time: June to November

Taste: rather inconspicuous, but gives mushroom dishes a colorful peppery taste

Risk of confusion: none, resembles the following edible purple ruby knight

Purple Ruby Knight (Lepista nuda)

Habit: 5 to 15 cm high, smooth, shiny, domed to funnel-shaped hat, with a flat, rolled-up edge when old

Hat color: bright violet, brownish with age

Stem: purple and bulbous with silvery-white longitudinal fibers

Slats: purple

Occurrence: beech and spruce forests, sometimes on meadows or on compost heaps

Collection time: September to November

Risk of confusion: none

Meadow mushroom (Agaricus campestris)

Growth habit: 10 cm tall, initially spherical, later flat hat, similar to the mushrooms in the shop

Hat color: gray-brown to white

Handle color: white

Slats: gray-pink, later dark gray to black

Occurrence: meadows, green areas, paddocks, grasslands

Collection time: May to November

Risk of confusion: poisonous carbol mushroom, unpleasant smell, chrome-yellow flesh in the base of the stem; poisonous white tuber agaric with white lamella

Winter turnip, velvet foot turnip (Flammulina velutipes)

Growth habit: 2 to 10 cm wide hat, thin-fleshed, with a greasy surface

Hat color: honey-yellow to reddish-brown with a dark center

Stem: ringless, velvety to felty, 3 to 8 cm long, yellow-brown above, dark brown below

Slats: white to pale yellow

Occurrence: on trunks and stumps of living or dead trees

Collection time: September to April

Flavor: tasty edible mushroom

Danger of confusion: poisonous pet with a smooth handle as the most important distinguishing feature

Special feature: even grows through a blanket of snow

Chapter 6

Nutrition and Health benefits of Mushrooms

Who says that fungus cannot do any good to your health? Mushrooms, though sometimes considered as vegetables are not really plants but fungi. What's interesting to note is that mushrooms are actually nutritious, too. In fact, they are called "functional foods" because they are low in all of those substances that the body does not need much of; fat, cholesterol, calories, and sodium.

For example, a cup of raw white mushrooms has a total of 15 calories, 2.2 grams of protein, 2.3 grams of carbohydrates and has 0 grams of fat. And though mushrooms come in different varieties, they pretty much have the same amount of nutrients per serving.

Improves Metabolism

Mushrooms are high in B vitamins like **thiamine** (B1), **riboflavin** (B2), **niacin** (B3), **pantothenic acid** (B5), and folate (B9). These B vitamins promote a healthy metabolism and lessen the risk of stroke. **Thiamine** is responsible for the production of new and healthy cells. It is often called the anti-stress vitamin because of its capability to fortify the immune system. **Riboflavin** is an antioxidant that helps the body in fighting free radicals or those particles in the body that cause damage to cells. This B vitamin slows the aging process and reduces the risk of heart disease. **Niacin** is known for boosting high-density lipoprotein (HDL) or the good cholesterol, which balances the bad cholesterol in the blood. **Pantothenic acid**, which is present in almost all food groups, is the vitamin responsible for the conversion of fats and carbohydrates into energy. Lastly, **folate** or **folic acid** is linked to having a good memory. It's also the vitamin responsible for the development of the fetus.

B Vitamins are responsible for promoting a better metabolism. This is because these vitamins help in the conversion of carbohydrates into glucose, which the body then burns to produce energy. Another role of B vitamins is metabolizing fats and proteins.

The Only Food With Vitamin D

Mushrooms are a good source of vitamin D. In fact, it's the only food that contains this critical vitamin. Humans stay under the sun to get vitamin D, and that's also what happens to mushrooms as they are exposed to sunlight. As a matter of fact, when mushrooms are exposed to ultraviolet B, that's when their sterol ergosterol is converted to vitamin D.

Boosts The Immune System

According to studies published by the American Society for Nutrition, mushrooms, particularly white button mushrooms, increases antiviral substances and other proteins that the cell releases when repairing and protecting the body. It also promotes the ripening of the dendritic cells found in the bone marrow, thus raising the defense against microbes that enters the body.

Serves As Antioxidants

Antioxidants are free radical fighting agents of the body. They help the body against dangerous oxygen molecules called free radicals. Antioxidants are mostly found among colorful vegetables but according to research, mushrooms like Portobello and crimini has the same oxygen radical absorbance capacity as that of a red pepper. White bottom mushrooms, on the other hand, were found to have a greater amount of antioxidants than that of tomatoes, carrots, zucchini, green peppers, or pumpkins. Antioxidants are linked to the prevention of cancer, heart diseases, and even Alzheimer's.

Contains Selenium For Bladder Health

Selenium is a rare mineral to find in one's diet but according to researchers, mushrooms are loaded with selenium, which is vital for bladder health. In fact, crimini mushrooms are an excellent source of selenium, 100 grams of raw crimini makes up 47 percent of your daily needs. Based on a published study in Cancer Epidemiology, Biomarkers & Prevention, a high level of selenium has a great impact on lowering the risk of bladder cancer. Selenium is also noted for improved immunity response to infections, enhances fertility among women, as well as reduces the risk of cancer and thyroid diseases.

Lowers The Risk Of Cancer, Diabetes, And Certain Heart Diseases

It's not only in consuming vegetables and fruits that we can prevent the development of dreaded diseases. A lot of studies have been made and proved that organically grown mushrooms, too can help lower the risk of obesity, diabetes, heart diseases, and cancer. It even helps nourish the hair and skin, as well as promote good weight management.

Anemia

People suffering from anemia are characterized by having very low levels of iron in their blood. This results in fatigue, headache, digestive problems and even reduced neural functions. Mushrooms are a cheap source of iron, which helps in maintaining a healthy formation of red blood cells in the body.

Cancer

Mushrooms contain compounds like lectins, glucans, proteins, and carbohydrates, which inhibits the development of cancer. According to research, daily intake of mushrooms can help prevent the possibility of breast cancers up to 60% among women. In another research, it has been found that mushrooms contain enzyme 5 alpha reductase that is linked to the prevention of prostate cancer among men.

Diabetes

Fiber diet among people with diabetes is vital. Fiber-rich diets can help type 1 diabetics to lower their glucose levels. The same diet can also improve type 2 diabetics to maintain good blood sugar, lipids, and insulin levels. This dietary fiber can be obtained from mushrooms. In fact, just a cup of grilled portabella mushroom or a cup of stir-fried shiitake has about 3 grams of fiber.

Heart Health

Mushrooms are also rich in potassium and vitamin C, which helps in improving the cardiovascular health. Blood pressure is regulated by the teamwork between potassium and sodium. Adding mushrooms to your diet will help you lower your cholesterol level, improve your blood pressure, and prevent you from any cardiovascular disease.

Some Other Things You Need To Know About Growing Mushrooms

Cultivating mushrooms could start only as an ordinary hobby. But if you'd like to make a business out of it, why not? If you are considering growing mushrooms for profit, why not invest on oyster mushrooms. Why oyster mushrooms? Oyster mushrooms are the easiest type to grow, and not to mention an exotic type of mushroom. Also, oyster mushroom can grow on just any waste products, straw, woodchips and coffee grounds to name a few.

In growing oyster mushrooms, you will need a dedicated area for growing the mycelium. Someplace where you can control the humidity, the temperature, the light, and other factors that may affect the growth of the mushroom. Also, make sure that your growing area is clean as this will prevent contamination. One way to keep your growing area clean is by following these simple tips:

1. When spreading the pasteurized straw to cool them down, do it in a clean environment. This can be done by washing down and disinfecting the surface to be cooled down.

2. Spray the air in the room with a 10% bleach solution.

3. Make sure to wash your hands diligently before handling the straw spawn and other substances that will be used.

If you'll keep the growing environment clean and make sure your oyster mushrooms are under the right weather conditions, you can expect to harvest oyster mushrooms of a good grade. And don't worry because just in case you are not able to sell them right away, Oyster mushrooms can also be preserved by drying them. Then, you can sell them even months from the time of harvest.

When selling your mushrooms, there are a couple of options:

At The Local Farmer's Market. This kind of event is a good avenue for people interested to buy locally produced products to crowd the market and can be a good opportunity for you to get regular consumers even. You can put up a small booth for you to sell your produce.

Directly To A Local Restaurant. You can also get regular customers by selling directly to a local restaurant. You may begin negotiating by offering samples of your mushrooms to a local restaurant's chef. Once he approved of the quality of your produce, that restaurant may end up as your regular customer.

Offering Them To Grocery Stores. Exotic mushrooms are popular and sellable nowadays. And just like restaurants, if a grocery store would want to buy Oyster mushrooms to sell to people, why would it not be from you? To be specific, try looking at upscale grocery stores whose customers would likely look for exotic mushrooms. What's more, a local grocery store might even give you the opportunity to demonstrate your produce and by doing so, you'll gain more customers for yourself.

Make Frozen And Pickled Oyster Mushrooms. If you have a large surplus of your Oyster mushroom harvest that you can't sell right away, another option to make a profit out of it is by making them into pickled mushrooms.

You may consider this pickled mushroom recipe:

You'll need:

- 1 pound fresh Oyster mushrooms, quartered
- 1 tablespoon pepper flakes
- 2 cups water
- 2 cups cider vinegar
- 3 tablespoons garlic, minced
- 2 tablespoons pickling spice
- 1 tablespoon salt

All you need to do is combine the second to the last ingredient and bring it to a boil in a large pot. Then, add in the mushroom. Cook until the mushroom is softened. Then, transfer to a jar. Then, cover and let chill for 10 to 12 hours.

Why Grow Mushrooms?

A lot of people think that mushroom farming takes great effort and that everyone is up for the task. But if you will into it, mushroom cultivation can be one of those things that you might want to include in your bucket list. It's one of those fun and eye-opening experience that you would not want to miss.

Whatever kind of mushroom you are aiming to raise, or wherever you want to grow it, there would be room to learn something from it. Just as mushrooms enrich the soil, you too will have an enriching experience should you decide to grow mushrooms.

Here are some of the reasons why one must consider growing mushrooms:

Growing Mushrooms Is Fun. Just like when planting any other plants, seeing those fungal formations grow and propagate will bring a sense of satisfaction for all your hard work. If you are the type of person you is ever inquisitive and observant of creating and seeing things develop, growing mushrooms just might be the right hobby for you.

Growing Mushrooms Is Educational. As was previously mentioned, mushrooms are not plants; they are fungi. And because of that simple fact, it would be impossible to grow mushrooms minus the learning. Cultivating mushrooms will open your mind to the contribution of fungi to the ecosystem. Because they are very different from plants, they require a different way to grow, and that requires for one to dig into the mushroom cycle life. Growing mushrooms is like devoting some quality time to an intricate science project.

Growing Mushrooms Teaches You To Be More Self-Sufficient. It's always a joy to grow your own food. Some plant their own vegetables. Others grow herbs in little pots. If you enjoy mushrooms, you don't always have to order in a restaurant or sweep the stalls of your favorite groceries to get some; you can grow them yourself. Wouldn't that be liberating? It gives you such a feeling of self-reliance.

Growing Mushrooms Will Save You Some Dollars. If you are thinking about spending for a mushroom kit as something, think of how much more you can save in the long run. Just look at it as an initial investment. Later on, the ROI can even be double, triple or even quadruple of that.

Growing Mushrooms Are A Sight To See. Mushrooms are beautiful. There are species that resembles flowers. Some of the mushrooms that are a sight to behold are Reishi, pink oysters, and shiitake mushrooms. If you enjoy looking at flower gardens and meadows, you would also enjoy looking at growing mushrooms.

Growing Mushrooms Expands Your Sense Of Taste. When you start to grow mushrooms, you will be very specific about them. You will begin to dig into recipes where each of those edible mushrooms is best with. What's the best dish to include oyster mushrooms? When you grow mushrooms, it will just blow your mind to know about all the sumptuous dishes you can make out of them.

Growing Mushrooms Allows You To Recycle. Mushrooms are not difficult to grow. If you have broken pots at home, any old cardboards or used coffee grounds, you can start growing mushrooms on them. This is not only helpful to the environment, but it also takes recycling to a brand new level.

Growing Mushrooms Sparks Interests. Everything that we are not used to seeing is fascinating. And because growing mushrooms cannot be compared to planting plants in a pot, it sparks interest and makes us more and more fascinated and curious. And if you are growing mushrooms, what's best than to know the answers to your questions about mushrooms from people who are also into the same hobby. Growing mushrooms is a worthy reason to meet people to share your knowledge with and gather info from.

Growing Mushrooms Gives You More Superior Ones Than Those Bought Elsewhere. Mushrooms that are homegrown are always the best. For one, they don't get stressed with the process of traveling from where they are harvested to which supermarket they would be destined to go. If you will look at mushrooms sitting on the shelves of a local grocery, the one that are home grown are always larger, fresher, tastier, and healthier. Growing your mushrooms yourself gives you the assurance that you are getting only organic ones, free from all those chemicals and pesticides that may even impose harm to your health in the long run.

Growing Mushrooms Open Your Mind To Having A Deeper Appreciation For Nature. Going mountain climbing, deep sea diving, snorkeling, visiting wondrous sights—all of these activities bring you closer to Mother Nature. That is the same effect that growing mushrooms can give you. You will get to appreciate their beauty, how they thrive in the wild and the mystery of how they grow. When you begin to study them, you will see them more in their natural setting.

You will get to see them in a brand new light. If you appreciate the rising and setting of the sun, or the waves as they hit the shore, or the birth of a puppy, or the blossoming of a rose, you will also appreciate how mushrooms grow.

Chapter 7

How to grow edible mushrooms at home

Cultivating Mushroom for food involves the production of human consumption edible mushrooms, which may be large or small. You will need to perform consumer research to understand market demand while increasing them for business. If the benefit of this crucial food commodity is not known to your potential market, a lot will be considered; in terms of marketing strategies to inform about the uses of the product. The shiitake, Oyster mushrooms, white, Enoki, and Shimej are cultivated in different types of edible mushrooms. The white mushroom is the most grown type, and some are fleshlier and thicker in different sizes. The growing of mushrooms depends on the species you choose; certain types are quite good, and most people prefer.

You need a nursery with suitable temperatures, usually moist, to grow them. Mushrooms will not rely on sunlight to develop, unlike green plants; therefore, they can grow in damp, dark areas. Their development will only take a couple of days to see progress. Cultivated mushrooms have a spontaneous growth that starts overnight, but normally takes a couple of days to develop. We are increasing in two phases of the pin phase accompanied by the stem size increase.

Ways to grow mushrooms: depending on your needs, you can grow mushrooms in different surfaces. You need a large space to grow edible mushrooms for commercial purposes, but cultivation for home use is on small surfaces that you can do on your own. Thus you can use:

Growing area perfect for commercial production

Office files that can be rendered at home.

Ware cabinets or moist bins

Cultivating mushrooms is a great effort because they make good food in gourmet restaurants and hotels. These provide the vegetarian meals with a nice garnish and are rich in vitamin B and essential minerals such as copper and potassium. If you get a good market supply like hotels and grocery stores, field mushrooms like the Oyster, Morels, shiitakes, and portabella will give you a good amount of money.

Steps to Cultivate Mushrooms: However, remember the temperature and water conditions of the climate to get the most out of your cultivation. Humid, it's perfect past dark conditions. This cheap project would involve in their good condition a few seedlings in the form of field spore seeds. Take the following steps to get them to grow:

Prepare for planting

A 2-inch deep growth field. Fill the bed with smooth soil and straw (optional fertilizer)

Test the bed's humidity level that should be roughly 95 to 100 percent

Sprinkle the offspring with wet cloth and fill with

Give the spores to grow for two to three weeks

As they grow the stem and cap separate to maturity, so you can harvest them. Using nitrogen material for the optimum natural growing of the mushrooms; it will provide you with healthy-looking forms in exchange for more quantity and quality.

How can I produce champignons? Oyster Mushroom Cultivation: An Easy and Good Way to Get Started China is the top oyster mushroom producer in the world, but more people are finding out how easy it is to cultivate their own. The growing of Oyster mushrooms is a rewarding experience. Once the production area is properly set up, the gardener simply needs to perform some basic repairs to facilitate healthy growth of the mushroom.

It is possible to make a mushroom garden indoors or outdoors. The process of establishing an oyster mushroom garden includes choosing oyster mushrooms for cultivation, setting the position of the container or greenhouse, and preserving the mushrooms. The gardener will pick a bunch of mushrooms attached to a stem base while picking oyster mushrooms from the grocery store for propagation.

A handful of wet wood shavings such as pet bedding should be put in a thin, damp brown paper bag to plan the initial step of oyster mushroom cultivation. The mushrooms were produced from the base of the plant. Cut off the base of the stem and place it in the bag of wet paper. Fold carefully over the top of the bag and place another wet paper bag inside that contains wet wood shavings as well.

You can also fold this paper bag and put it in a plastic container. The bottle should be stored for three months in the fridge crisper. The mushroom stem sprouts during this period and is ready to start a mushroom garden at home.

Once the base of the mushroom has been growing for three months, it is important to arrange bedding for the mushroom plant. The surface is called the substance in which the mushrooms are to develop. In a ten to one mixture of water and peroxide, one way is to sterilize wool. In the peroxide solution, the handle should be moisturized. Then a plastic freezer bag and some mushroom base can be applied by the gardener.

Fill the container with straw and mushroom base alternating sheets. Out of the container should be squeezed some extra peroxide vapor. It is necessary to keep the bag at room temperature. The gardener should slice a small x or small holes in the bag once the inside of the bag turns white with mushroom seeds. The mushroom is going to bloom in the bag's hole. Most gardeners of mushrooms enjoy hanging a bag in the kitchen and picking up mushrooms while they bake.

Many people prefer to use coffee grounds or sterilized sawdust instead of grass. Diluted peroxide should be used to sterilize whatever surface is desired. Several people may be susceptible to the spores of the production of the oyster mushroom and prefer to keep the bags outside or in a shed instead of in the home. The mushrooms do their best in dark places that are kept at about 70 degrees.

Growing mushrooms at home

Many people just buy their magical mushrooms, before, but picking them from the wild is another alternative. But some enterprising magical mushroom fans cultivate their own in the home. We are going to examine this latter option.

Most mushroom cultivators begin with Psilocybe cubensis as it's the most common and also the easiest to grow. There are many distinct methods to begin growing mushrooms, however, we will only look at a single fundamental method.

Psilocybe cubensis

All methods start with a single important component: the spore. A spore develops into one mushroom, and a mushroom could create thousands and thousands of them.

Spore prints, along with being used for identification of uncontrolled mushrooms, may likewise be utilised to nurture mushrooms. The spores that are dry on the print has to be hydrated to be used.

Sterility is significant in all facets of mushroom growth; bacteria or mould are able to prevent them from growing completely but might also cause polluted mushrooms to emerge.

Many mushroom growers buy spore syringes (full of spores and sterile water) from providers instead of creating their own.

The cost of a spore syringe can range from $10 to $20 based on the specific strain.

Magic Mushroom Spore Syringe (magic-mushrooms-shop.com)

The brown rice is blended with the water along with vermiculite to make a loose, fluffy noodle cake, a nutrient-rich surrounding where the mushroom spores will probably develop.

The substrate is then placed in the jars that can be sealed and sterilized together with the pressure cooker or canner.

The spores must start to grow in a week and generally seem like principles of white fuzz known as mycelium. If mould develops, or nothing happens, then something went wrong.

If the cakes have been covered in mycelium, they are placed into the plastic container to start maturing.

When removed from the container, the cakes need to acquire mould and a great deal of humidity.

If all goes well, mushrooms start to develop after a couple of weeks and are ready to decide when the caps start to grow up. Each cake may create mushrooms for as much as a month, typically in waves.

A lone cake can create countless mushrooms. They could decompose pretty fast; therefore, mushrooms are often dried or refrigerated to maintain them.

Growing mushrooms is not all that pricey but getting the spore prints or spore syringes can be challenging since it is not necessarily legal to purchase, sell, or have them.

How to Start Your Own Mini Mushroom Farm in 5 Steps

I'd love to see all the more small-scale mushrooms farmers out there carrying top quality mushrooms to their neighborhood. In any case, I'm mindful it can feel somewhat overwhelming with many areas to learn. To help, I've composed a diagram of the 5 fundamental advances you'd have to take and some valuable tips to begin:

Find some space

Most indoor spaces can be adapted for use, yet perhaps the most ideal approach to move toward this is by asking what kind of space do mushrooms need to develop? The 3 main stages of the mushroom-growing Cycle indicates that there are 3 principal stages to the developing procedure, each requiring a different space:

Stage 1: Mixing and Inoculation - where the substrate ingredients and mushroom planting structures are mixed and packed away (more on this procedure in a moment)

Stage 2: Incubation - where they develop bags are left in a warm dark space for the product to grow all through the bag

Stage 3: Fruiting - where the colonized bag is presented to outside air, mugginess and a little light which makes the mushrooms 'natural product'.

Out of the various stages, stage 3 is the trickiest to make, however positively feasible for a great many people to undertake for under $1000. I've manufactured a couple of various fruiting room plans throughout the years, yet our latest one is the least expensive and easiest, worked inside a hydroponics cultivation tent like this one.

The size of the space you need relies upon lots of variables like what number of mushrooms you're meaning to develop, how you build your fruiting room and what choices you have accessible to you. You might not have any desire to invest in this if you're taking a shot at your very own project however, as it's a great deal of work. As a guideline, it'll take you around 10-15 hours/week to develop 10kg mushrooms on a normal week after week cycle.

The fundamentals are simply access to water and electricity, and adequate air ventilation for the cultivation space. We were given free utilization of a 125m2 space in a place of business directly in the center of a downtown area, which is where the UK's first Urban Mushroom ranch is based.

You could also utilize space in basements, garages, barns, shipping compartments. Somebody we know is, in any event, considering growing mushrooms in an old disused toilet block!

No doubt about it, she's reasoning that the disabled room would make an ideal mixing room, with the men's an incredible hatching room, and the ladies a perfect spot for the mushrooms to grow product; pure genius!

Decide on your design

When you have a thought of where you may base your small-scale mushroom ranch, you can begin to imagine what your farm may resemble - it's the ideal opportunity for a plan.

Incubation

The picture above shows the primary Incubation room I worked in that's inside a shipping compartment. That's right, simple shelving in a protected room! This works superbly for littler packs, and are frequently utilized for Shiitake or small-scale Oyster cultivation. You can also utilize hanging rails rather, similar to the picture below, in case you're developing Oyster mushrooms in greater section bags:

Oyster mushroom mycelium developing on coffee grounds in 12Kg hanging segment packs

Contingent upon where you're based, you may require a warming or cooling framework set up to keep the temperature around 20 - 24C, so having a protected space will downplay vitality use.

Fruiting

There are numerous opportunities when it comes to making your fruiting room – and I will share a couple of ways it very well may be finished. There are ups and down to every one of these alternatives, and it's hard for me to state which one would be best for you, as it relies upon your space and budget. In the event that you join our free email course (below), you'll get the opportunity to become familiar with why we think the hydroponics tent is an incredible choice for a great many people who are starting out.

Build your farm

When you've settled on your structure, it's a great opportunity to focus on and build it. There's a great deal of detail for this stage, with an abundance of topics to cover in any helpful manner in this article, however, it's absolutely do-capable for the vast majority even without to your skills. Eric (who I run GroCycle with), and I are entirely essential at DIY, and we assembled this little 5m2 fruiting room rapidly and effectively in several days.

At the point when we manufactured our greater Urban Mushroom Farm arrangement, we did a portion of the work ourselves and just asked a companion who was a builder/carpenter to assist with the rest. The fact of the matter is, if you need to do it, you can get it going. It's not advanced science, and it should also be possible on a budget initially and gradually improved in case you're shy of assets.

Start Growing (The Low-Tech Way)

How about we imagine for a minute that you've presently made the spaces for your small-scale mushroom ranch and are prepared to get developing. Low-tech mushroom developing is a technique we've been dealing with within the course of the most recent couple of years which doesn't require the huge, costly and energy-intensive equipment regularly utilized in commercial mushroom cultivation.

Typically, the substrate ingredients (frequently straw or sawdust) are warmed to high temperatures so as to pasteurize them and kill off any competing living beings. Low-tech strategies sidestep this progression or discover low energy approaches to accomplish a similar result.

For instance, we develop Oyster mushrooms on coffee grounds (effectively purified from the brewing procedure), sawdust pellets (effectively sanitized from the heat made during their generation), or straw (effectively sanitized by absorbing a high pH cold water shower). Waste coffee grounds are an abundant (and right now purified) asset. Different features of the low-tech approach include utilizing quickly developing, forceful strains, and by utilizing higher spawn rates than are ordinarily utilized in enormous mushroom farms.

Oyster mushrooms are by a long shot the simplest, to begin with, and can be developed dependably with significant returns utilizing low-tech techniques. For more data on developing Oyster mushrooms, look at our top to bottom step by step guide for developing Oyster mushrooms here.

In the course of the most recent few years, we've been trialing different varieties in utilizing the low-tech approach also. Most other gourmet varieties so far have delivered mixed outcomes, yet through bunches of analyses, we're presently having solid and great accomplishment with Shiitake mushrooms - one of the most exceptionally prized gourmet varieties.

Shiitake mushrooms - developed utilizing simple low-tech strategies

I'm certain with more experimentation different assortments will be mastered soon too. It's also simpler to learn. At the point when I initially began developing mushrooms, I needed to learn definite research strategies so as to get predictable outcomes. Presently you can gain understanding of the nuts and bolts in a couple of hours and be effectively developing right from the beginning.

Harvesting and Selling your mushrooms

Picture that your first bags have colonized well and in the following 2-3 weeks you put them in your new fruiting room. You watch little mushroom pins show up and later develop, multiplying in size each day until they are golden mushrooms and prepared for you to gather. You place them in a plate, alongside other perfectly shaped mushrooms, and start contemplating who will get the opportunity to appreciate them at their best.

Look at the deal cost per kilogram for Oyster and Shiitake mushrooms in your nation, by perceiving the amount they're sold for in any of the above spots that you can discover them in. The value you can get will differ in every nation.

In the UK for instance, privately developed new Oyster mushrooms can sell for around £10 (US$13) per kg and Shiitake at £15 (US$19) per kg. In Australia, Oysters bring a noteworthy AU$ 40 (US$ 29) per kg! You would prefer not to try to compete with modest imports, so you're expecting to offer just to places that will acknowledge (and pay) for the quality you offer.

Aside from local freshness and high quality of the mushrooms, you have other selling focuses as well: your mushrooms are privately developed utilizing manageable strategies. Lots of gourmet specialists, shoppers, and retailers esteem these sorts of things and will support you by addressing an excellent cost.

More income?

Obviously, selling crisp mushrooms isn't the main way you can profit from your efforts. For anybody keen on transforming it into a regular of low-maintenance income, there are bunches of different methods to earn money, while spreading the marvel of the mushroom world as well. Different approaches to profit with mushrooms:

Mushroom developing units: delivering bags that help individuals to develop their very own mushrooms at home can be an incredible source of additional salary. They make extraordinary gifts and can help spread the news about your business as well.

Workshops, visits, and courses: when you've mastered the developing procedure, you can run courses and short workshops training individuals what you do and why mushrooms are incredible!

Street nourishment/celebration slow down: take your mushrooms to a week by week food market or to celebrations and cook them in a wide range of delicious approaches to include additional worth. A wide range of individuals who love mushrooms will love what you present!

Mushroom based snacks: You can include additional incentive by transforming a portion of your yield into mushroom burgers, tempura or croquettes - impeccable healthy veggie snacks.

Partnership with social enterprises/charities working with burdened groups: developing mushrooms is an extraordinary movement to stall out in and utilize your hands, just as learning a wide scope of different skills. Connect with an association working with ex-prisoners for instance and get subsidizing to help instruct them to develop mushrooms!

85

Chapter 8

Common problems in growing Magic Mushrooms

When you've requested your underlying syringes of spores or fluid culture, it's a great opportunity to begin pondering what you'll have to do when they show up.

For all intents and purposes each system, from setting up your substrate to the last fruiting procedure, should be performed in conditions that are as sterile as could be expected under the circumstances. You currently realize that, at its center, developing mush-rooms is a race between the mycelium you're attempting to develop and different life forms that will attempt to pollute your way of life. The best substrates for mushrooms are additionally the best substrates for some different sorts of molds and microorganisms, which can and will repress mycelial development.

The objective is to develop out your mycelium as fast as could be expected under the circumstances, before any contenders get an opportunity to grab hold. To give your mycelium the ideal possibility, you'll need to wipe out or limit wellsprings of defilement in your home, and make the cleanest working conditions you can.

Keep It Clean

As an at-home mushroom cultivator, you should attempt to keep your home as perfect as conceivable constantly. This implies no filthy dishes getting mildew covered, no stale nourishment in your trash transfer, no residue on your knickknacks, every one of the alcoves and crevices in your restroom free of shape, etc. All these potential wellsprings of contaminants can wreck your difficult work and cause issues well into what's to come.

Regardless of how clean your home might be, you've seen residue and contaminants it. The residue that courses through your house is made out of human skin cells, garments strands, plant dust, and an assortment of different substances, including contagious spores. These airborne form spores are one of the essential wellsprings of defilement in your tasks.

Each house is unique. A few people may have homes sufficiently clean to enable a large number of these procedures to be performed on the outside, including agar moves. Others think that its difficult to take a perfect spore print anyplace in their home. Numerous components influence home neatness, including the year the house was developed, the structure materials that were used, the home's history, (for example, flooding), the kind of HVAC framework, etc.

At the point when I start my work in the kitchen or the cleanroom, the clean zone where I do my development work, I think about all the residue that happens normally noticeable all around. If I bring something into my sterile work region from outside, it should initially be disinfected, regardless of whether it has just contacted the air — as you currently know, air is a long way from sterile.

At whatever point you get another apparatus or move your hand to snatch something, inquire as to whether the development you're making may make defilement. The equivalent goes for different surfaces: if it's feasible for the residue to develop on a surface, you should sanitize it if you intend to take a shot at it or contact it. For instance, I generally re-clean my gloves if I snatch a bit of paper towel from outside my work zone, if I modify my seat, or if I scratch my face.

Build up A Cleaning Protocol

Before you start any mushroom-developing undertaking, think about finding a way to clean your home. You might not need to follow up on every one of these proposals; it relies upon your individual conditions.

Before You Start

- Clean your home all through; mop and residue

- Shampoo covers at any rate once

- Wash all mats or consider evacuating them for all time

- Clean the cooler

- Keep the trash transfer perfect and flushed of nourishment

- Pay unique thoughtfulness regarding alcoves, cran-nies, and corners in restrooms (high dampness = increasingly chance for molds)

- Do not let junk sit inside; keep a top on trash

- Remove indoor plants (soils contain unfortunate organisms)

- Dust roof fans

- Change bed materials routinely

- Keep pet territories and beds clean

- Caulk broken windows

- Keep shoes at the entryway

- Do not work in covered rooms, or think about laying plastic

Get ready to Work

- Focal air, climate control systems, fans, and so forth.

- Clean surfaces with a 10:1 arrangement of water to fade, Lysol, isopropyl, or comparative cleaner

- Shower; wash hands

- Wear clean garments

- Work on a hard, smooth surface

- Do not deal with the floor

- Run air purifiers in your work region

- Have dust covers and hairnets accessible for use

Continuous

- keep trash transfer clear of nourishment

- Remove terminated nourishment expeditiously from the cooler

- Vacuum routinely, yet never just you fill in as it kicks up particles

- Dispose of tainted containers early

- Never open defiled containers inside

Know Your Enemies

At the point when you develop mushrooms, you are endeavoring to make ideal conditions for the mushroom mycelium you're spreading. Tragically, those conditions are likewise ideal for some other organisms that we call contaminants. The most well-known contaminants in mushroom development are molds (which are parasites also) and microorganisms. If these contaminants interact with your substrate, they'll develop reasonably quickly, regularly quicker than your mushroom mycelium.

Issues with defilement are the essential explanation individuals quit any pretense of developing mushrooms. It very well may be exceptionally unsettling to need to discard a whole clump of containers that you went through hours making up, or a whole rack of housings that you went through a month preparing. Propelled cultivators' experience less defilement than fledglings since they can spot potential tainting early and cure the circumstance before it can spread. Figuring out how to spot potential contaminants early is the most ideal approach to guarantee accomplishment in your tasks and avoid future issues.

Molds

Molds can show up in a wide exhibit of hues — dark, green, yellow, dim, pink — in your containers. There are many, numerous sorts of molds that you may experience in mushroom development. Here are the absolute most regular ones.

Blue-Green Mold (Penicillium spp.) There are several species in this variety, and most are difficult to differentiate without the utilization of a magnifying lens. The blue-green shape that shows up in your activities could be similar species used to make the anti-toxin penicillin. Under a magnifying instrument, distinguishing proof of the class is genuinely simple in view of the long chains of conidia (spores) that structure on a fanned base, yet similarly as with numerous kinds of shape, recognizable proof of the real species can be an errand, in any event, for somebody prepared in the field.

This form is incredibly normal for the home mushroom cultivator, so the primary concern you have to know is that it regularly shows up as a green or pale blue green settlement. This state is normally not uncommonly quickly developing, yet if you notice it in any containers, they ought to be disposed of right away. I have seen mushroom mycelium totally wrap a state of blue-green shape, yet that doesn't mean the settlement is dead. If you somehow happened to separate the container and move it, you would spread the contaminant all around the following period of your task, and it would most likely fall flat. This shape is most ordinarily found in containers of colonizing grain. Likewise with most contaminants in grain containers, there is little any expectation of sparing the substrate. It ought to be tossed out right away.

Green Mold (Trichoderma spp.)

Trichoderma (trike-goodness derma) is one of the quickest developing molds you're probably going to experience. It's most ordinarily connected with packaging layers, however it can likewise influence containers. I've additionally observed it showing up with some consistency in straw ventures. In nature, there are around 30 types of this form, most generally found in the dirt and on dead wood.

Trichoderma regularly shows up as mycelium when it's young. At this stage, it's a brilliant white mass of shape, however as it ages, it turns an intense green. Green implies that the settlement has started to shape and discharge its spores, so it ought to be evacuated right away. With a touch of understanding, you ought to have the option to differentiate between the white of a youthful trichoderma settlement and the white of mushroom mycelium. By and large, mushroom mycelium is wispier and not as thick, particularly while it's as yet colonizing. Trichoderma regularly shows up as a strong white settlement, without obviously recognizable rhizomorphs or mycelial strings. Trichoderma is the essential shape related to the annihilation of agaricus crops on business mushroom ranches. A considerable lot of these ranches use fungicides to keep this shape from showing up in the peat greenery of the packaging layers.

There aren't generally any compelling approaches to battle this form once it has started to sporulate, particularly if it builds up itself in a colonizing container or sack. Expel the debased undertaking from the rest when it's spotted. If you discover green form in a packaging layer, it might be conceivable to evacuate the tainted bit and spare the remainder of the packaging.

Spider web Mold (Hypomyces spp., Cladobotryumdendroides or Dactyliumdendroides)

One of the most widely recognized contaminants for mushroom cultivators, web shape is regularly discovered developing on cakes or packaging layers. It's practically indistinguishable from mushroom mycelium, which makes it extremely hard to recognize. There are a few highlights you can figure out how to search for that may assist you with spotting it early. To begin with, spider web form is some-what grayer than the unadulterated white of mush-room mycelium. Second, it has a wispier development propensity than mushroom mycelium. At long last, it will in general develop a lot quicker than mushroom mycelium. It can develop from a little spot on the packaging layer to a softball-sized disease in only several days.

If this form develops close to creating mushrooms, it can colonize and slaughter them too. If you distinguish it early, you can use hydrogen peroxide to battle it Aspergillus spp.

93

While most shape your experience in mush-room development is not especially pathogenic to people, aspergillus is a special case. If you breathe in aspergillus spores in enormous amounts, you may get an infection known as aspergillosis. At the point when con-fined to the lungs, manifestations can incorporate hack, trouble breathing, and chest torments. If the malady advances into the body, it can cause issues including the lungs and kidneys.

Aspergillus species can frame a wide range of hues in a settlement, including dark green, yellow-green, or dark. As a result of the wide scope of morphology and the trouble of appropriately recognizing the species, take incredible consideration when working with and discarding any shape you experience, and abstain from taking in huge amounts of any spores.

Lipstick Mold (Geotrichum spp.)

As the normal name recommends, this form gets its name from the pinkish shading it procures as it ages. The main time I experienced this form was in PF containers when I initially began developing. While not especially normal anyplace but rather in

PF containers, it's a simple contaminant for the apprentice to distinguish. If you experience this shape in your containers, you have to rethink your sterile system.

Bacterial Contaminants

Microscopic organisms can likewise be a critical issue in mushroom development. Microscopic organisms regularly show up as a reasonable or grayish ooze, generally joined by a sweet or impactful smell. Here are two of the most widely recognized microscopic organisms in mushroom development.

Wet Spot (Bacillus spp.)

Most generally present on grain bring forth, this bacterium shows up as a reasonable, grayish sludge on the grain in the container and produces an impactful scent. Mushroom mycelium won't colonize territories of the grain that are contaminated with microbes. Bacterial endospores are a typical issue with produce creators, as they may not be murdered during an ordinary disinfection cycle. In case you're having issues with microscopic organisms, consider using the splashing strategy for your grain, increment your cleansing occasions, or both.

Bacterial Blotch (Pseudomonas spp.)

This is one of only a handful not many ailments that influences mushrooms after they have begun to shape. Some of the time the mushroom tops will seem to have spots and are decaying before the tops themselves are full grown. This is brought about by bacterial contamination. The spots may initially seem vile, and they in the long run structure noxious injuries on the mushroom. If you experience this sickness on mushrooms that are framing, expel the tainted mushrooms right away. You ought to likewise diminish the moistness in your developing condition and increment the measure of approaching natural air.

Tainting is an unavoidable truth for the home cultivator or business producer.

It's ideal to stay hopeful, yet set aside the effort to thoroughly consider all your disinfection methodology and attempt to decide how the pollution happened. Each cultivator learns by experimentation, and the blunders are frequently more educational than the triumphs, as they can assist you with avoiding botches on future, bigger clusters of mushrooms.

Discarding Contaminants Because a few molds can be unsafe for your wellbeing, and most can be inconvenient to your development ventures, never open tainted containers inside. Opening containers inside just spreads the shape spores around your home, releasing the potential for future tainting. After you open the containers, discard the substrate outside. At that point put on something else before going anyplace close to your lab and developing zone. Shape spores adhered to your garments can be followed back inside with you.

If a container has a genuine measure of defilement, and you need to spare the container, consider pressure cooking the container before you open it. This will murder all the form spores inside and keep them from spreading. Opening a container that has a great deal of defilement will frequently bring about an obvious haze of spores being discharged. If the entire container is green (or some other shading) and you would prefer not to pressure cook it before opening it, simply toss the whole container out. Sparing one container does not merit the potential for contaminants long into what's to come.

After you have dumped out the defiled containers, wash them out with a hose outside before you bring them back inside. When the containers are back inside, wash them out with cleanser and water.

Using a Glovebox

Keeping your home as spotless as conceivable is just a little piece of the race against molds and microscopic organisms. Despite the fact that the air inside might be cleaner than the air outside, it's not almost clean enough for a considerable lot of the methodology used in mushroom development. To perform them effectively, you'll need some gear explicitly made to deliver situations clean enough for sterile work: a glovebox or a stream hood.

A glovebox is a fixed or semi-fixed box that makes a clean, still-air condition around the materials with which you're working. Spores and different contaminants settle out of the air to the base of the container, leaving you with sterile air to work with.

While not an ideal arrangement, a glovebox is an extraordinary minimal effort alternative that will build your odds for progress.

Gloveboxes are regularly utilized by apprentices for methods, for example, making syringes and fluid societies, vaccinating containers, and grain moves. At any rate, I would prescribe the formation of a basic glovebox preceding your first develop. It will get you into the propensity for receiving sterile systems and will at last be advantageous to your endeavors. The following best technique is the development of a stream hood, however that requires a genuine venture of time and cash, and I don't suggest it until you have a few become added to your repertoire.

Numerous varieties of the glovebox can be made, contingent upon your individual needs. One variety that I would not suggest, in any case, is the expansion of a HEPA channel unit to your crate. A few people cut an opening into the side of the glovebox and connect a HEPA channel/fan unit, ordinarily accessible at tool shops. There are two principle reasons why I accept this is a poorly conceived notion. To begin with, it crushes the essential objective of a glovebox — to make a still-air condition. Consistent wind stream into your glovebox will make whirls of contaminant particles in the case and around your work. At the point when you open containers, these twirling contaminants will be considerably more liable to get in.

Second, while HEPA channels are intended to clean air with 99.98 percent productivity, the units' outlet ports are not enough fixed. They regularly permit the presentation of defiled air into the outlet stream after the channel. I have not experienced any promptly accessible air channel units with channel lodging seals that are reasonable for glove-box work. If it's not too much trouble remember this when you think about glovebox structures.

Make an Inoculation Room

When you've made a glovebox, you'll need a detached spot to utilize it. The perfect spot for an in-home immunization room is prob-capably a storeroom. I set up a table in a room wardrobe for the clean work of my first develops. Storage rooms have a few focal points over different pieces of the house. Almost still-air situations, storerooms are generally secluded from the air-flow frameworks in the remainder of the home, and they for the most part have entryways you can near keep away from incidental air flows. If your storeroom is covered, it's ideal to lay some plastic down over it to constrain the measure of residue you kick up at whatever point you enter. Additionally make certain to take off any garments, towels, and other comparative things from the storage room. Garments will in general harbor contaminants, which are discharged at whatever point the garments are moved or bumped.

It's additionally conceivable to immunize bumps in a spotless washroom without the utilization of a glovebox, if your home has a generally low spore tally. Washrooms generally have tile floors as opposed to covering, so the measure of residue in restroom air is typically lower. Additionally, washrooms as a rule comprise of hard, smooth, sturdy surfaces that are anything but difficult to clean with rock solid cleaning items. The fundamental downside of washrooms is their moistness, which urges molds to multiply. I lean toward storage rooms to washrooms for vaccinations and other cleanroom work, with or without a glove-box. Be that as it may, if a storeroom isn't accessible, the washroom is the following best alternative.

Whichever room you decide to utilize, tidy up all surfaces in the live with an answer of 10:1 water to fade, isopropyl liquor, Lysol, hydrogen peroxide, or another appropriate cleaning item. Numerous individuals likewise decide to splash air sanitizers in the room.

Chapter 9

Equipments and Supplies

Pressure cooker

The pressure cooker is probably the most essential piece of equipment in your mushroom cultivation arsenal. You'll be using it regularly as an autoclave to sterilize substrates and equipment. You can buy them from grocery stores, second hand stores, scientific shops and mushroom supply stores. Both new and used models are advertised online.

The choice of make and size will depend largely on what you can afford, but there are some critical considerations to take into account:

Much of its use will be for sterilizing substrate in quart-sized mason jars. So buy one that's at least big enough to hold 6–10 jars.

It should preferably have a steam release valve or "stopcock" that you can control rather than a "rocker" type that automatically releases steam if the pressure goes above a certain level. The rocker type can lead to very rapid release of pressure and steam and is likely to cause anything liquid in the pot to boil up and overflow. This can be very messy and you can lose most of your material. What you really want is for the pressure and steam to reduce naturally once the pot has been removed from the heat source. This should take about an hour and a half. It must also retain a vacuum while it is cooling, so non-sterile air cannot get in to contaminate your cultures or substrate.

There must be an accurate dial to show internal pressure.

Buy from a reputable source. Look for models that have a minimum number of parts that can wear out–and where you can buy spares if you need to.

Pressure cookers can be very dangerous. They can explode if the pressure gets too high. They can implode if you pour cold water over them to cool them down. It is easy to scald yourself with the steam. So safety rule number one is to read the manual and know exactly how to operate your pot.

Make sure that it is working properly, with the lid properly sealed and locked into place. A bit of Vaseline on the rim will help to keep the lid sealed.

Use a basket inside the pot so that whatever you put into it doesn't touch any of the surfaces. You can make a basket, using galvanized steel wire. Stand the basket on a rack or trivet to keep it out of the water. Anything standing in water is not being sterilized as the pressurized steam cannot reach it.

There should be at least half an inch of water at the bottom of the pot. Some pots may give an amount in cups that should be used. Some of the water will evaporate in steam, and you want to be sure that there is enough left to maintain the pressure for the required period.

Depending on the heat source you are using, check to see whether your pot can be used on a gas burner or only on a stovetop.

Heat the pot slowly and let it cool down slowly. Doing this too fast can lead to the glass inside the pot shattering.

Let a full head of steam develop before you close the stopcock.

Never leave a pressure cooker unattended. Know how to operate the emergency release according to the manufacturer's manual.

Never put a sealed container into the pot. Make sure that there is a way for air to escape through the lid.

Finally, to ensure sterile conditions, wrap the outlet of the stopcock with an alcohol-soaked cloth prior to opening the valve. This will ensure that no spores or other contaminants enter the cooker when you vent the steam.

Most bacteria and other microorganisms are killed if you leave them in the pot for 15 minutes with the pressure at 15 PSI and the temperature at 121°C/250°F. Specifics about times required for different substrates are provided in later chapters.

Alcohol lamp or mini torch

You will use the flame from these items for sterilizing equipment like inoculation loops and scalpels while you are working. Alcohol lamps are filled with rubbing alcohol and capped with a cotton wick and metal cap. Mini torches are generally butane-based. They are used by chefs and for soldering small items, so they are fairly easily available. They are easier to use if they have a base and can stand upright on the table top. Alcohol lamps can be found at scientific or mushroom supply shops.

Mason jars, lids and filter discs

These are three items, but are used together. You are going to use the jars to create spawn–ie the mixture of substrate and mycelium that can then be moved to other locations to propagate mushrooms.

You want plastic lids because you want your jar sealed, but air must be able to escape so that the jar does not explode in the pressure cooker. To modify them, cut or drill a 1-inch hole in the center. Then, fit the lid with a filter disk so air can enter, but harmful contaminants are blocked.

The filter disc is made of a synthetic fiber that can be sterilized and re-used. If they discolor from contact with substrate or mold spores, soak them in a quarter-strength bleach solution. You can buy the discs pre-cut to fit your lid, or make your own.

The pre-cut ones that are sold specifically for mushroom cultivation are very effective, with some being sold with the same specifications as HEPA air filters – i.e. 99,97% effective against microbes as small as 0.3 microns. They can be re-used multiple times.

For a cheaper option you might want to make your own using Tyvek–this is the material used for indestructible mailing envelopes. You can buy it in building supply stores. Just note that filters made from Tyvek should be cut larger than the lid and placed **over** the lid, not between the lid and the mouth of the jar. It must be tied down with elastic bands or the regular screw top outer band. Some people will place it between two lids that have had holes cut in them at the same position. The whole will meld into one piece once it has been heated in the pressure cooker. Use these discs only three or four times and then discard them.

Chapter 10

Indoor Cultivation

In a dry or winter atmosphere, growing mushrooms inside is frequently the main choice. Mushrooms can be grown inside all year. Albeit growing inside can require more work, it delivers the best mushrooms and yields.

If you are looking for extra or full time pay, an elective method to plant during the off season, or explicit nourishing or restorative advantages, growing mushrooms inside may be your answer.

Growing mushrooms from a minor perspective isn't troublesome once you are equipped with the information on how mushrooms grow and their needs.

Mushrooms are straightforward animals that grow in obscurity with some stickiness. Mushrooms can be grown inside in any atmosphere and in any season and almost anyplace with the correct conditions, including storm cellars and creep spaces, just as other littler spaces like condos. In contrast to plants, these growths are one of just a couple of life forms that grow without chlorophyll. They get all their sustenance from the material or substrate they grow in or on. A substrate can be straw or wood chips.

You need a growing room where you can control the temperature. Your growing room ought to keep up a temperature of 78 degrees

Fahrenheit (25 degrees Celsius). You additionally should have the option to control the stickiness and the light.

Tidiness is additionally basic to solid mushroom growth, as there are variously conceivable sullies that can damage or demolish mushrooms. Purifying the substrate or straw is an incredible beginning for dispensing with conceivable taints. All growing region surfaces and apparatuses ought to be cleaned with a 10% fade arrangement before including the substrate. Wash your hands unfailingly and completely before you handle your produce, substrate, or devices.

There are supplements that can be added during the growing procedure to improve flavor and increment yields, including soy, cottonseed and horse feed dinner.

Mushroom packs

Mushroom packs are accessible with prepared to-vaccinate bring forth. These packs accompany spores and every one of the provisions expected to begin growing. The least difficult mushroom growing units incorporate a sack of sawdust or straw that has been immunized with produce.

Packs incorporate full guidelines and some have plastic tents for controlling humidity. Fundamentally, you discover an area that is room temperature and away from any immediate daylight for your arrangement and substrate. At that point you shower fog a few times each day for stickiness.

The following part subtleties the diverse culinary mushroom types that are mainstream for home producers that incorporate cremini, oysters, shiitake, wine tops and portabellas, yet there are more.

Making Money Growing Mushrooms

At the point when you get familiar with the craft of growing mushrooms, you may choose to grow for benefit. Gourmet mushrooms are a significant yield, despite the fact that you ought to have your market set up. Where you can sell will rely upon the amount and kinds of mushrooms you grow, just as your area. As customer request has expanded as a consciousness of the medical advantages has a cover. The market for mushrooms is better than anyone might have expected and restorative mushroom inquire about is supporting the interest for more species.

Mushroom growing can be fulfilling and productive. The obstruction to section is more information than cost as costly gear isn't required. Be that as it may, there is an expectation to absorb information. Timing can be fairly precarious, and certain species involve extraordinary administration.

Gourmet mushrooms are getting a charge out of a growing prominence. This expanding request has made gainful open doors in any event, for little indoor cultivating with the colorful mushrooms, for example, oyster and Shiitake mushrooms.

Oyster mushrooms are a gourmet mushroom that is productive for the home producer because of interest and the low cost hindrance to growing. The oyster mushroom grows rapidly and a home cultivator can create around five harvests every year, even in their extra time of as meager as a couple of hours out of each week.

Because of the way that oyster mushrooms are so productive, even a little space can create great pay. Truth be told, a growing region of around 100 square feet can create as much as 2,500 pounds of mushrooms a year! In a region as little as 500 square feet, around 12,000 pounds of mushrooms can be grown and harvested every year. At the point when retail costs for oyster mushrooms are at about $6 per pound, which they have been, that compares to a gross salary of $72,000 every year.

Your odds of achievement can significantly increment with the information picked up from this book, just as an anomaly and enthusiasm for organisms.

Selling Mushrooms

Since new mushrooms bring the most cash and sell the best, you need to sell your mushrooms when you harvest them at whatever point conceivable. Any mushrooms you don't sell can be solidified or dried to sell later.

Be set up early to advertise your mushrooms. Find out about any ranchers' business sectors that are inside a sensible separation of your area. These business sectors can draw huge groups, including the business sector and eatery proprietors just as different purchasers. These can be extraordinary contacts and you could have responsibilities from purchasers for your future harvests before you even start growing.

Eateries search for extraordinary and nearby produce; mushrooms are no exemption. Make the rounds in your general vicinity and meet café proprietors. Give them free examples and let them realize your collect calendar.

Markets and some wellbeing nourishment stores stock mushrooms and numerous likewise acknowledge nearby cultivators. If you can supply them with new gourmet mushrooms, you probably won't require some other clients. You can inquire as to whether you can set up a free example table for a day to take into account their clients, too.

The Future of Mushrooms

Individuals are getting taught about the medical advantages and culinary attributes of mushrooms. The request is expanding. Growth innovation keeps on progressing as filled by the interest. Research is being done to expand the time span of usability of mushrooms including bundling innovation and capacity, just as improving the mushrooms themselves, which will satisfy the need.

The investigation into the restorative advantages of mushroom likewise proceeds and new points of interest are found. This will likewise make request increment. The simplicity of delivering mushrooms taking things down a notch makes this an ideal pay open door for some individuals.

Chapter 11

Outdoor Cultivation

Mushrooms can be grown and cultivated outside on fertilizer piles just as on disregarded yards. Mushrooms love soils that are wealthy in natural issue. To construct a mushroom bed, you'll have to lift a 10-inch bit of turf and make a profundity of around 4 cms, ensuring that each square is around 60 cms separated. At that point, using a garden fork, release the soil underneath the turf squares and include a portion of your favored natural issue to make the soil rich. If your soil is poor, it's prescribed to use garden fertilizer or some well-decayed excrement. Maintain a strategic distance from the utilization of substance manures as these may not be great in advancing mushroom growth. When this is done, you can cover the mushroom generate daintily over the outside of the soil and mix it softly with the soil. Make a point to keep it pretty much 1 cms profound. At that point, put the turf squares back solidly. Ensure that the soil is kept oystermy. Note that when growing mushrooms outside, the climate condition is to be considered as this will direct the fruiting of the mushrooms.

Fertilizer

One famous growing mode for growing mushrooms outside is by setting up manure. The conventional strategy used in setting up a fertilizer is finished by mixing roughage in with creature compost. This kind of fertilizing the soil procedure is energized as it permits the engendering of microorganisms that assistants in the pre-processing of the natural materials in the soil will in the long run become nourishment for the mycelium.

In the initial segment of the fertilizing the soil, the material is turned and watered from time to time. Before the finish of the fertilizing the soil procedure, the warmth brought about by the procedure of disintegration is urged to collect as this washed away a portion of the overabundance alkali and slaughters excluded bothers in the soil.

Mushroom treating the soil is used to make a uniform material. Be that as it may, for bigger manure generation scales, it would require a ceaseless progression of crude materials and some taking care of hardware and the best possible ability. Today, the greater part of the manure offices are undermined as a result of our biology concerned society with regards to keeping up a smell free and contamination free treating the soil generation.

Tips For Harvesting Your Mushrooms

You'll realize the mushrooms are prepared to harvest when the tops are completely discrete from the stems. Consider what opening an umbrella resembles, when your mushrooms resemble a completely stretched out umbrella they are prepared to accumulate.

It is a poorly conceived notion to select your mushrooms starting from the earliest stage, wind them from the base until they are isolated from the growing material. The least demanding path is to cut the base of the stem with a blade.

For mushrooms grown on logs, harvesting is basically the equivalent - getting the mushroom at the base of the stem and marginally turning them away from the log. In the wake of harvesting, the logs will at present keep on growing more natural products until the fourth week. You have to enable a few months for the mycelium to recover from the collect and afterward recover. At that point, you may deliver another yield should you wish to. Note that a similar log can at present be used and remains beneficial up to its sixth year.

Chapter 12

How to store mushrooms

Proper storage extends shelf-life. The best method for long-term storage is to dry your harvest and then store it in an airtight container in a cool, dark place.

Freezing after drying (if done correctly) could keep the mushrooms fresh for an infinite amount of time.

Store Your Mushrooms for an impressive period of time by dehydrating Them:

Drying out mushrooms in a dehydrator is a mind-boggling approach to store a wealth of mushrooms. You can use this system to ensure that the privately gained mushrooms in your cooler don't ruin before you get around to eating them.

Try not to use mushrooms that are already beginning to dry out or get spoilt. Signs that your mushrooms have started rotting include ooze storing up superficially, wrinkly, shriveled mushrooms, mushrooms that get darker or get dim spots, or you see any awful stench originating from the mushrooms.

About Dehydrating Mushrooms in a Dehydrator

Most mushrooms dry flawlessly, not just holding anyway in any event, getting flavor simultaneously. Precisely when rehydrated in high temp water, the surface is practically indistinguishable from that of fresh mushroom. Dried mushrooms can be used within a year.

Even though mushrooms can be dried in the broiler, you get the best results if you use a dehydrator following this simple method.

Cleaning and Slicing Mushrooms

To start, you have to clean the mushrooms. Contrary to legend, raw mushrooms don't retain lots of water during a quick wash. Try not to skip washing them in water. Try to get all the dirt off the mushrooms with a vegetable or mushroom brush.

A comprehensive cleaning makes your cooking prep a lot easier, particularly with mushroom types that have lots of alcoves and crevices, for example, maitake mushrooms.

Depending on which is least demanding for the state of the mushrooms, either clean them entirely and afterward cut them or the other way around. It is adequate to cut them first and after that perfect them if that appears to be almost effortless.

Cut the mushrooms into pieces that are between 1/4 to 1/2 inch thick. The thicker the cuts, the more it will take to dry, so consider this when you are cutting.

Using the Dehydrator

Arrange the cleaned, cut mushrooms on the dehydrator plate, ensuring that none of the pieces touch or cover. This permits the best wind stream around them, and they will dry quicker and evenly. If they contact or cover, a few territories may hold some dampness.

114

Dry the cut mushrooms at 110 F until the pieces are firm dry (or follow the explicit rules that accompany your dehydrator). This methodology takes 4 to 6 hours for 1/4-inch cuts and as long as 8 hours for thicker cuts.

Allow the dried mushrooms to cool totally before removing them.

Putting away and Rehydration

Move the cooled, dried mushrooms to glass compartments and spread immovably with tops. Name the containers with the substance including the type of mushroom and the date of drying. Store the containers from direct light or warmth.

If you are favored with an abundance of fresh morel mushrooms, drying them is an extraordinary way to maintain these springtime treats so you can enjoy them all year.

Morels dry perfectly, holding the majority of their flavors. When suitably dried and rehydrated in boiling water, their surface is practically indistinguishable from fresh morels. Dried morel mushrooms can be put away inconclusively since they are not exposed to dampness.

Steps for Dehydrating Morel Mushrooms

Even though morels can be dried in grills or even before a fan, you will get the best results if you use a dehydrator.

Clean and Soak the Morels

In any case, clean the morels. Disregard all that you've found out about not washing mushrooms in water, and give these fortunes a decent flushing off. You may need to slice the morels down the middle the long way to make cleaning them easier.

Creepy crawlies every now and again alcove in the honeycomb-like precipices of these mushrooms, even after the flushing off. To dispose of them, break down around 2 tablespoons of salt in a half-gallon of water. Dip the morels in the salt water for about 10 minutes, yet not longer than 30 minutes. While there is a great deal of persuasion out there about soaking them in the salt water medium-term, don't do it. Morels lose its quality and their surface isn't as great with prolonged soaking.

When the morels have had their douse, give them another wash to dispose of the salt. Delicately smash the mushrooms in a clean dish towel to get free of excess water as could be expected.

Sort or Slice the Morels

Even though morels can be dried whole, you need the mushrooms to be uniform in size when they go into the dehydrator with the goal that they dry uniformly.

You can do this by stacking each dehydrator plate with equal-sized morels: the plate of morel mushrooms will be prepared to leave the dehydrator sooner than the plate of bigger ones.

On the other hand, cut bigger morels into parts or littler pieces with the goal that they are nearer to the size of your humbler ones.

Place them on the Dehydrator Trays

Arrange the morels on the dehydrator plate, ensuring that none of the pieces contact or cover.

Dry the Morels in the Dehydrator

Dry them at 125 F (52 C) until the pieces are firm dry. This will take 4 to 6 hours for little slices and as long as 8 hours for bigger or whole morels.

Cool the Dried Morels and Transfer to Glass Jars

Allow the dried morels to cool completely before moving them to the glass holders.

Pour out the water, saving the lavishly enhanced fluid for soup stocks and sauces.

Mushroom Equivalents, Measures, and Substitutions

Convert estimations of mushrooms, from fresh to dried, and canned to cups

Mushrooms add a sublime richness to dishes, and with the numerous varieties open, bring intriguing surface, flavor, and appearance to a recipe. When cooking with mushrooms, regardless, your formula may require this fixing cut, estimated in cups; in any case if you are buying whole mushrooms, by which method will you get the amount to purchase? The beneficial thing is, with a couple straightforward changes, you will have the option to choose what number of whole mushrooms are in a cup of slashed, similarly as a couple of various reciprocals.

Mushrooms are one of those fixings that are offered in a wide scope of structures: whole, direct, canned, and powdered. So when cooking a dish that uses mushrooms, there's an average possibility you might not have the right kind of mushroom your formula calls for.

If you like mushrooms and will cook with them frequently, remember you'll generally have mushrooms close by if you stock canned mushrooms, dried mushrooms, and powdered mushrooms in your storeroom.

Conclusion

For anyone interested in agriculture, be it as a hobby or as a means of earning a living, mushroom growing is an extremely viable option. Popular as a delicacy and food source, growing mushrooms while it is profitable can present some problems for the grower. One of the biggest features is the fact that the fungus is very sensitive to environmental changes and extremely prone to infection. Excessive contact with cultivators can affect the plant and thus crop yield. The only option left to a farmer to ensure that crop yield is good and adequate for his purpose is to automate the whole process of mushroom growing. This can be achieved by proper use of the fungal equipment. Mushroom tools can relate together to a variety of tools. The most important tools for mushroom growing include mushroom growing, mushrooming, compost processing, tunneling, mushrooming, and mushroom growing. Depending on the need, one or the other type of mushroom tool must be selected to increase the yield of the mushrooms. When choosing the right fungal equipment, it is often difficult to choose the right equipment that best suits your needs. As with most other machines, it is safe to trust numbers. The most popular mushroom equipment is probably the best on the market. To make sure that the mushroom equipment you buy at the time of purchase is the best possible brand, it is a good idea to gather background information before actually spending your money. Search for success stories on different mushroom equipment brands and choose the ones with the best ratings. Among other things, the right equipment is, of course, the key to the success or failure of a potential mushroom harvest. However, the right equipment does not just depend on the brand you choose. To decide exactly which brand is best for you, you should also consider the size of your business. The larger a farm, the more technologically advanced mushroom equipment they would ideally need. Ultimately, however, it would be advisable to choose, especially for commercial farmers, equipment that helps to produce "good quality" specialty mushrooms.

CPSIA information can be obtained
at www.ICGtesting.com
Printed in the USA
BVHW042318080621
609012BV00003BA/585